Progress in Orthopaedic Surgery

Vol. 4

Joint Preserving Procedures of the Lower Extremity

Edited by U.H. Weil

Contributors

J. U. Baumann, Basle · H. Judet, Paris · J. Judet, Paris
P. Maquet, Liège · R. Schneider, Biel · A. Schreiber, Zurich
K. Schürmann, Basle · H. Wagner, Nuremberg/Altdorf

With 87 Figures

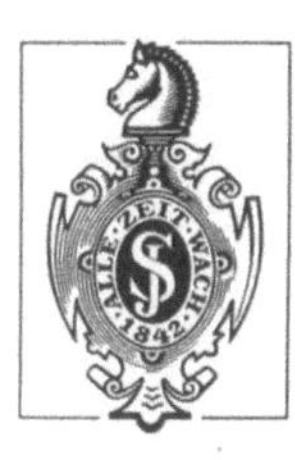

Springer-Verlag
Berlin Heidelberg New York 1980

Editor: Ulrich H. Weil, M.D.,
60 Temple Street, New Haven, Connecticut 06510
USA

ISBN-13: 978-3-642-67536-2   e-ISBN-13: 978-3-642-67534-8
DOI: 10.1007/ 978-3-642-67534-8

Typesetting: Fotosatz Service Weihrauch, Würzburg

2125/3321 543210

Contents

Preface

The fourth volume of Progress in Orthopaedic Surgery is somewhat different from previous publications of the series. The editors have again tried to present two topics but the publications presented from the European literature are of very recent origin.

In the age of total joint replacement it was felt to be imperative to counteract the present tendency to treat every joint which does not seem to be healthy with an artificial replacement. Orthopaedic surgery seems to be influenced by trends. In 1963, E.A. Nichol discussing intracapsular hip fractures, quoted from Alice In Wonderland in an editorial written for volume 45B of the Journal of Bone and Joint Surgery "The Queen had only one way of settling all difficulties, great or small, "Off with his head"!". Today one could paraphrase his implied critizism by saying "Out with the joint". No one doubts that joint replacements have been of great value in treating degenerative joint changes, but it is already apparent that replacement operations are not the ultimate answer for treating every joint deformity.

This volume represents the European experience of different types of surgery in treating arthrosis of the joints of the lower limb. A reader of the Anglo-American literature will find suggestions in it which reaffirm his uneasiness in considering only one solution for problems concerning lower limb joints. I feel strongly that there are other ways which allow a patient to function well with less extensive operations. Alternate methods are published in this volume and it behoves us to reconsider these well documented procedures. The papers by H. Wagner, J. and H. Judet, A. Schreiber, R. Schneider and P. Maquet represent some of the European experience in dealing with these problems.

I do not believe that Dr. H. Wagner requires an introduction to Anglo-American readers. His work on leg length discrepency correction is already a classic in orthopaedic literature. For many years he has investigated joint preserving operations of the hip joint. His "mini" reconstruction of the hip joint is a solution which, if properly applied, will prevent more extensive operations. His latest experiences are transmitted in the lead article of this volume.

The volume contains two publications on gait and on lower extremity bracing of patients suffering from myelomeningoceles in addition to joint preserving operations of the lower limb. Dr. J. U. Baumann and his staff are some of the foremost investigators in central Europe in researching gait and its abnormalities. Anyone who has visited his institute realizes how important his contributions in this field are to orthopaedics.

New Haven, Connecticut October 1979   Ulrich H. Weil

Resurfacing of the Hip Joint

H. Wagner*

Among the large variety of structural and functional problems affecting the hip joint there are many which require surgical treatment because of the magnitude of the pain. On one hand, the classical conservative osteotomies of the proximal femur or the acetabulum can no longer be expected to offer help in these cases. On the other hand, the relatively young age of the patients prohibits the indiscriminate use of a total hip joint replacement. This is where, with our present day knowledge, the resurfacing procedure may fill the gap in the therapeutic armamentarium of the hip surgeon. It preserves the hip joint by merely replacing the articular surfaces with polyethylene, metal or ceramic implants (Fig. 1A).

Compared with total hip replacement, the resurfacing procedure offers as its most outstanding advantage a greater ease of conversion to alternative procedures should these become necessary. The preservation of the bone stock of the femoral head and neck circumvents a number of the disadvantages inherent in total hip replacements.

Due to its asymmetrical shape the proximal end of the femur is subject to bending forces under physiologic loading and cycling. These torque forces are transmitted through the trabecular structures of the head and neck, and are absorbed by the compression trabeculae medially and the traction trabeculae laterally (Fig. 1B). The stresses of the compression and tensile forces are easily handled by living bone. The total femoral endoprosthesis replacing the respected femoral head and neck lacks this natural mechanism for transfer of forces. Bending forces are therefore transferred directly to the stem of the prosthesis anchored in the medullary cavity. With the difference in elastic modulus between trabecular bone and the solid metal implant, the transmitted forces cause micromotion at the interface. With the passage of time this micromotion leads to bone resorption. The mechanical situation is such that a total hip prosthesis can almost uniformly be expected to fail with time. Violation of the intramedullary cavity increases the risk of infection and makes the treatment of an established infection significantly more difficult. Filling the medullary cavity with polymethylmethacrylate can release sufficient polymerization heat to cause thermal damage to the bone tissue. The resurfacing procedure avoids all of these problems which are of particular significance when dealing with younger patients.

---

* Orthopädische Klinik Wichernhaus, Surgeon-in-Chief: Prof. Dr. Heinz Wagner, D-8503 Altdorf/Nürnberg, Federal Republic of Germany

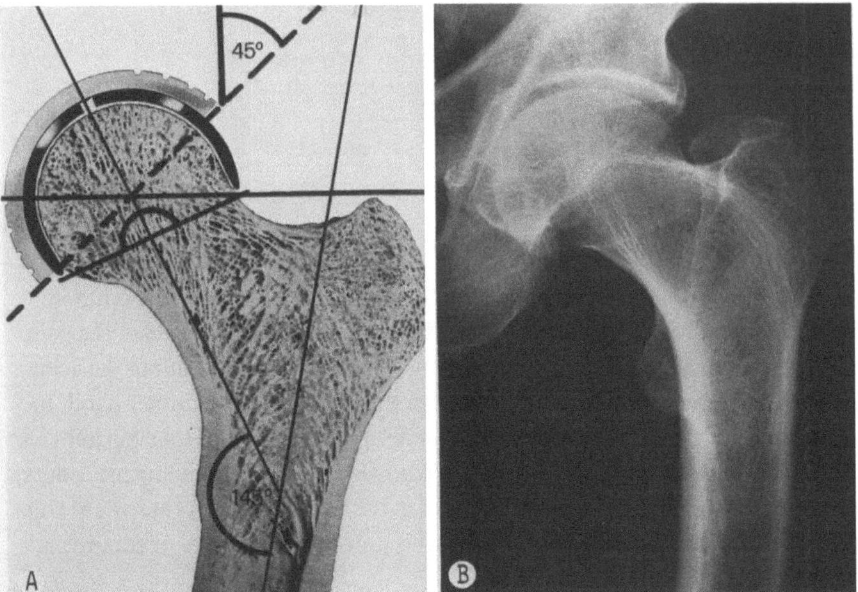

Fig. 1. A Coronal section of a model of a resurfacing prothesis. The polyethylene acetabular component should be inclined 45° and anteverted 25°. The cup for the femoral head is placed in valgus with respect to the femoral neck so that a perpendicular bisector of its base forms a 145° angle with the shaft of the femur. Through sufficient removal of bone stock from the medial segment of the head, the femoral cup is placed far enough laterally to cover the unreamed bony surface of the lateral head-neck junction. **B** Bony trajectories of the proximal femur. The compression trabecular system is relatively centrally located in the area of the head-neck junction. The traction trabecular system courses through the lateral portion of the femoral neck. It has to be preserved during reaming of the head

Experiments with homologous transplant of femoral and acetabular joint surfaces, were started in 1966 and first reported in 1968. They lead to the development of the resurfacing hip prosthesis. The resurfacing prosthesis was first implanted in 1974.

The prosthesis [1] consists of thin-walled hemispherical cup-shaped implants whose surfaces correspond in size to the normal cartilage surface of the hip. The resurfacing prosthesis is available in three standard sizes of 42, 46, and 50 mm, measuring the outside diameter of the femoral component. Two special sizes are available, a 38 mm model made in response to surgeons from East Asia and South America for their patient populations and an extra large 54 mm diameter model. It should be mentioned that these two special sizes are rarely required in western patient populations. Emphasis must be placed on the match of the prosthesis to the normal anatomical structures in the individual patient. Choosing too small a prosthesis makes the insertion technically easier but excess bone must be sacrificed from the femoral head. On the contrary, choosing too large a prosthesis makes the surgical procedure more difficult and requires excess reaming of the acetabulum thus weakening the medial wall and inviting stress fractures at a later time.

---

[1] Manufacturer of the prosthesis and instrumentation: Aesculap, D-7200 Tuttlingen, Federal Republic of Germany

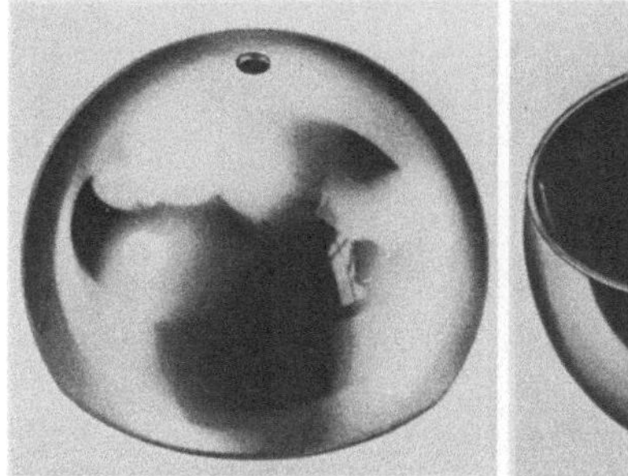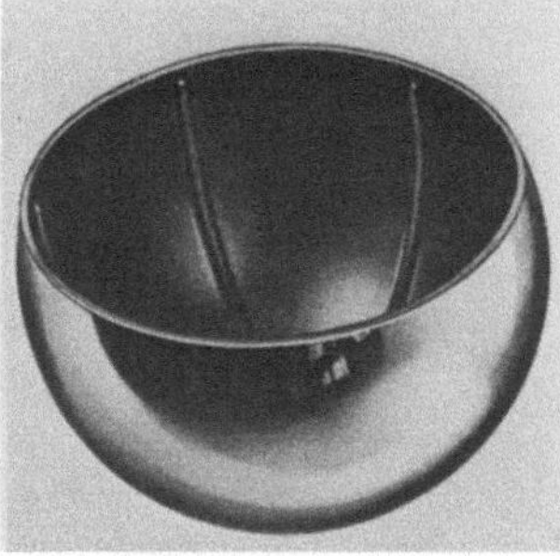

Fig. 2. The metal femoral resurfacing component of Co-Cr-Mo alloy. The central aperature allows air, blood, and excess cement to escape during insertion. The radially oriented ridges on the rough inner surface allow better cement fixation

The femoral component replacing the articular surface of the femoral head (Figs. 2 and 3) has a wall thickness of 3 mm and its outer surface encompasses 230°, i.e. its rim extends 25° beyond the equator of the joint. A centrally placed aperature allows the escape of air, blood, and excess cement during implantation. Two varieties of femoral components are available, one a Cobalt-Chromium-Molybdenum alloy and the other an aluminum-oxide ceramic.

Both varieties of femoral components are rigid implants to accommodate the relatively rigid structure of the femoral head. The subchondral trabecular pattern of the femoral head is vertically oriented with respect to the joint surface, as is the case with all convex joint surfaces. These rigid bone ends tolerate surface replacement with rigid implants since both respond to stress with only minimal deformation. This is of considerable importance to the longevity of the prosthesis since shearing forces are negligible on the femoral side of the endoprosthetic joint at the bone cement interface.

To gain better cement fixation, the metallic femoral component is manufactured with a lightly roughened inner surface and radially oriented ridges (Fig. 2). The inner aspect of the ceramic components cannot be produced with ridges for technical reasons and, therefore, has multiple small circular indentations for the cement fixation (Fig. 3).

The resurfacing prosthesis has the additional advantage of easy removal without sacrificing bone stock should this ever become necessary. This is of special importance if

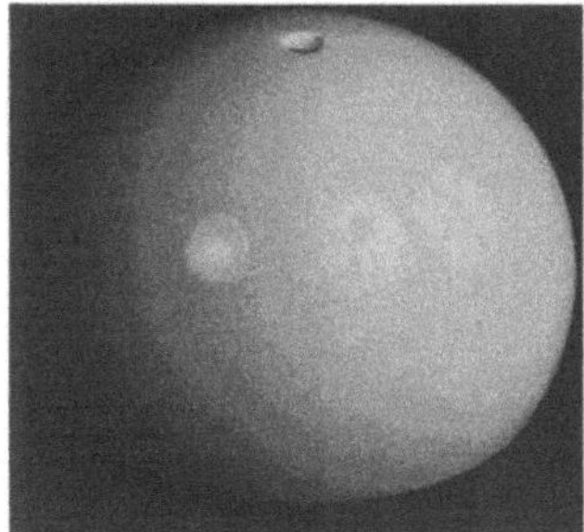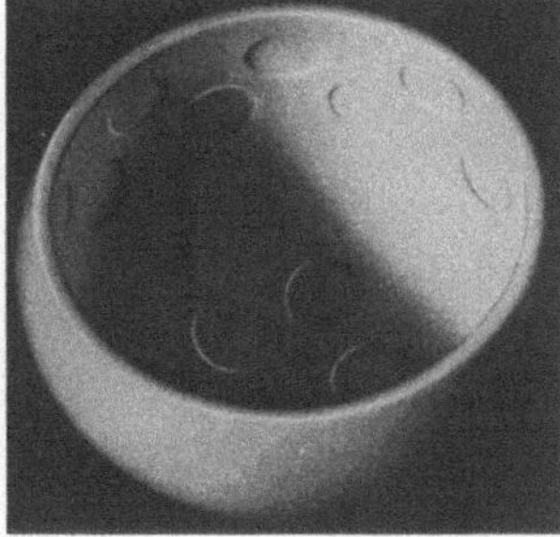

Fig. 3. Ceramic femoral head components of aluminum oxide (Rosenthal-Biokeramik). The inside and outside diameters are the same as for the metal components and also have the central aperature. The inner surface is rough and has numerous indentations for better cement fixation

H. Wagner

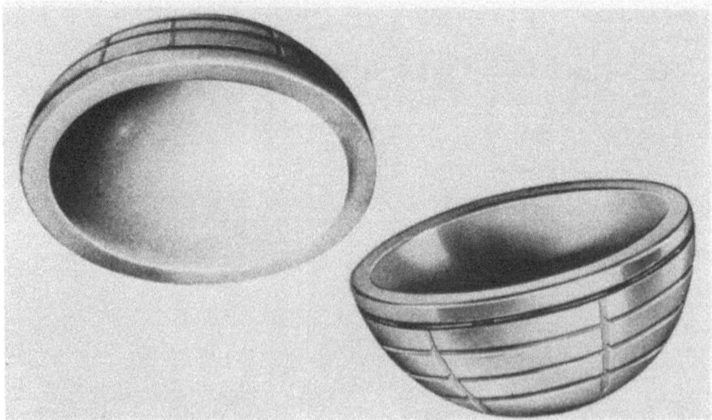

Fig. 4. Polyethylene acetabular component. Circular and radially oriented grooves on the outer surface of this 4 mm thick component permit better cement fixation. There is a radiopaque marker wire in the outer groove

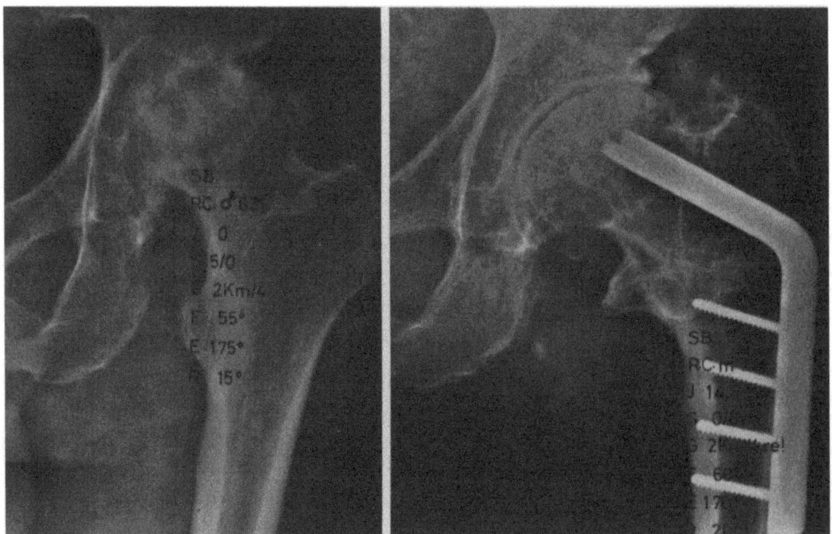

Fig. 5. Typical radiograph of a resurfacing prosthesis.
A Advanced coxarthrosis in a 55 year old female with acetabular dysplasia and subluxation. **B** Four years after resurfacing endoprosthesis

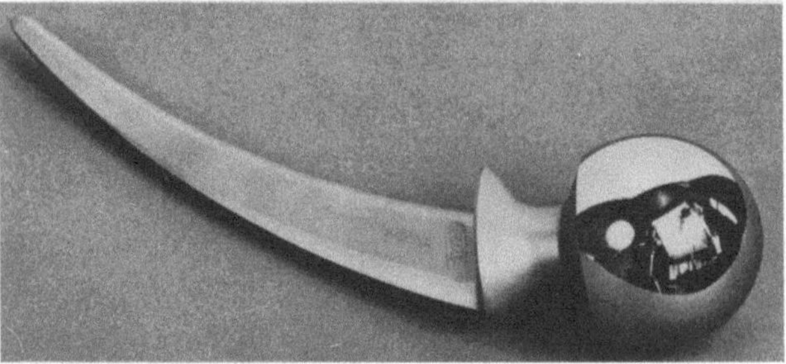

Fig. 6. Femoral endoprosthesis with the same head diameter as the femoral resurfacing component

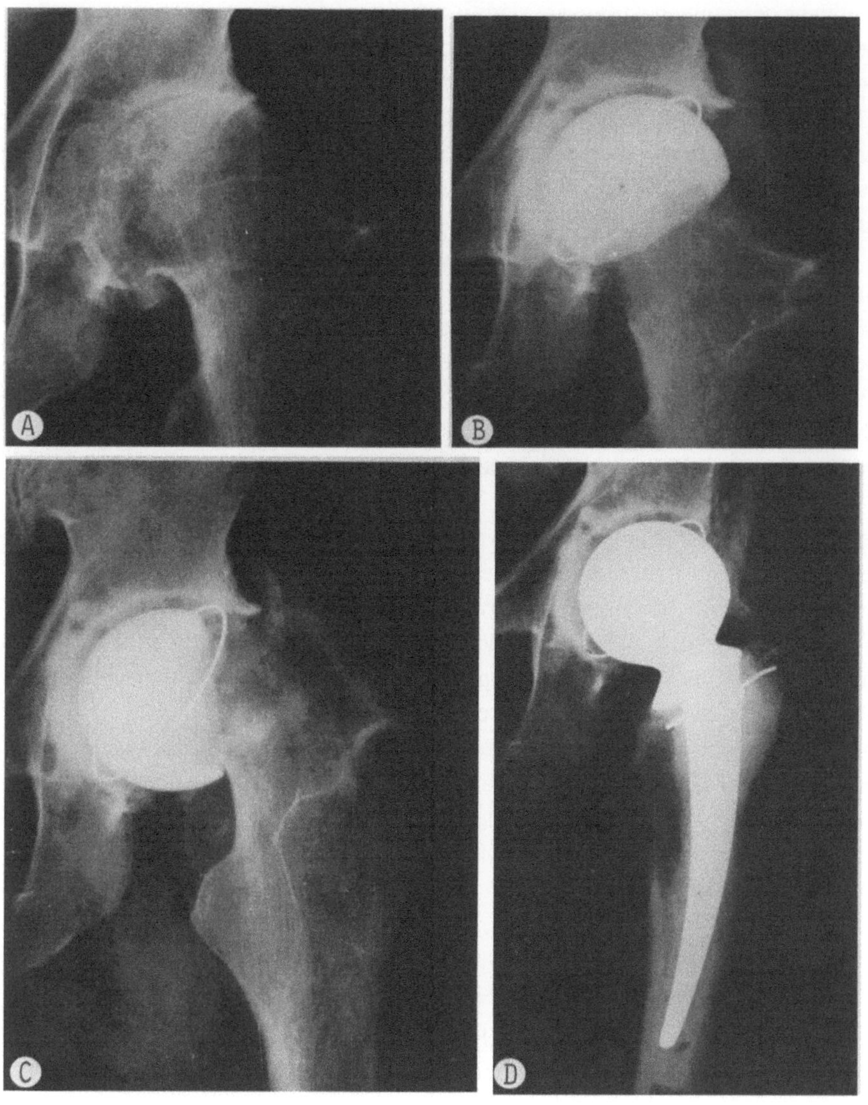

Fig. 7. Conversion of a resurfacing prosthesis to a femoral head replacement following femoral neck fracture. **A** Advanced coxarthrosis in a 57 year old male. **B** Three weeks after surface replacement. **C** Subcapital fracture of the hip four weeks after the resurfacing procedure. **D** Three months after conversion to a total hip replacement

removal of a firmly cemented component is required because of malposition or infection. Due to its radially oriented anchoring ridges, the metal cup can be elevated from the cement by a few blows against its rim. The cement base that remains can be fragmented with an osteotome and removed in pieces. A metal cup with transverse anchoring ridges or a sintered inner surface could not be removed from the cement without sacrificing the femoral head, an obviously great disadvantage. The ceramic component is removed by fracturing it with blows around its rim and then removing the fragments.

It has yet to be determined if there are significant clinical differences between the metal and ceramic components. Because of its microstructure and physical hardness characteristics, the ceramic component has a smooth surface which probably causes less wear on the polyethylene acetabular component. An additional advantage of the ceramic implant is its radiolucency which enables radiological evaluation of the underlying bone structure. Experience with the Co-Cr-Mo alloy is decades old and has been satisfactory. The ceramic implants have been used only a few years and it will be several more years before a final decision can be reached on which material is preferable for long term implantation.

The acetabular component replaces the articular surface of the pelvic side of the hip joint. It is a 4 mm thick high density polyethylene component whose depth encompasses only 175° and thus falls short of the equator of the joint. It has an inner diameter 0.1 mm greater than that of the corresponding outer diameter of the femoral component to allow tissue fluid lubrication of the joint. The acetabular component has a smooth inner surface and a convex outer surface with both circular and radical grooves for cement fixation. There is a marker wire along the rim to allow radiological monitoring of its position in the pelvis. Because of the relative thinness of its wall, the acetabular component is quite elastic and conforms to the stress deformations of the supporting pelvis. This elasticity combined with a preferably thin, somewhat elastic layer of polymethylmethacrylate may explain why radiolucent lines of resorption are rarely seen around the acetabular component following resurfacing procedures (Fig. 5).

Femoral component loosening or fracture of the femoral neck necessitates the conversion of the resurfacing prosthesis to a total hip prosthesis; requiring no disturbance of the acetabular component. Femoral endoprostheses with conventional femoral stems and with head diameters equal to those of the resurfacing femoral components are available (Figs. 6 and 7).

Disadvantages

The use of the anterior approach to the hip joint might be construed as a relative disadvantage since it requires more experience, more care, and greater attention to detail from the surgeon. However, if performed correctly this approach is superior to others. The bony fixation of the prosthetic components with polymethylmethacrylate demands a higher degree of perfection than is necessary in the total hip replacement. The cement surface contact area is smaller than that of a femoral endoprosthesis with a long intramedullary stem. This is of prime importance when dealing with the subchondral bone stock that has undergone atrophic changes. Exact positioning of the femoral component is required for optimal stress tolerance of the supporting bone.

Indications

An indication for surface replacement exists in any painful disease of the hip which is (1) refractory to nonoperative therapy and thus demands surgical intervention to correct the severe disability, (2) beyond the stage where the classical joint conserving osteotomies

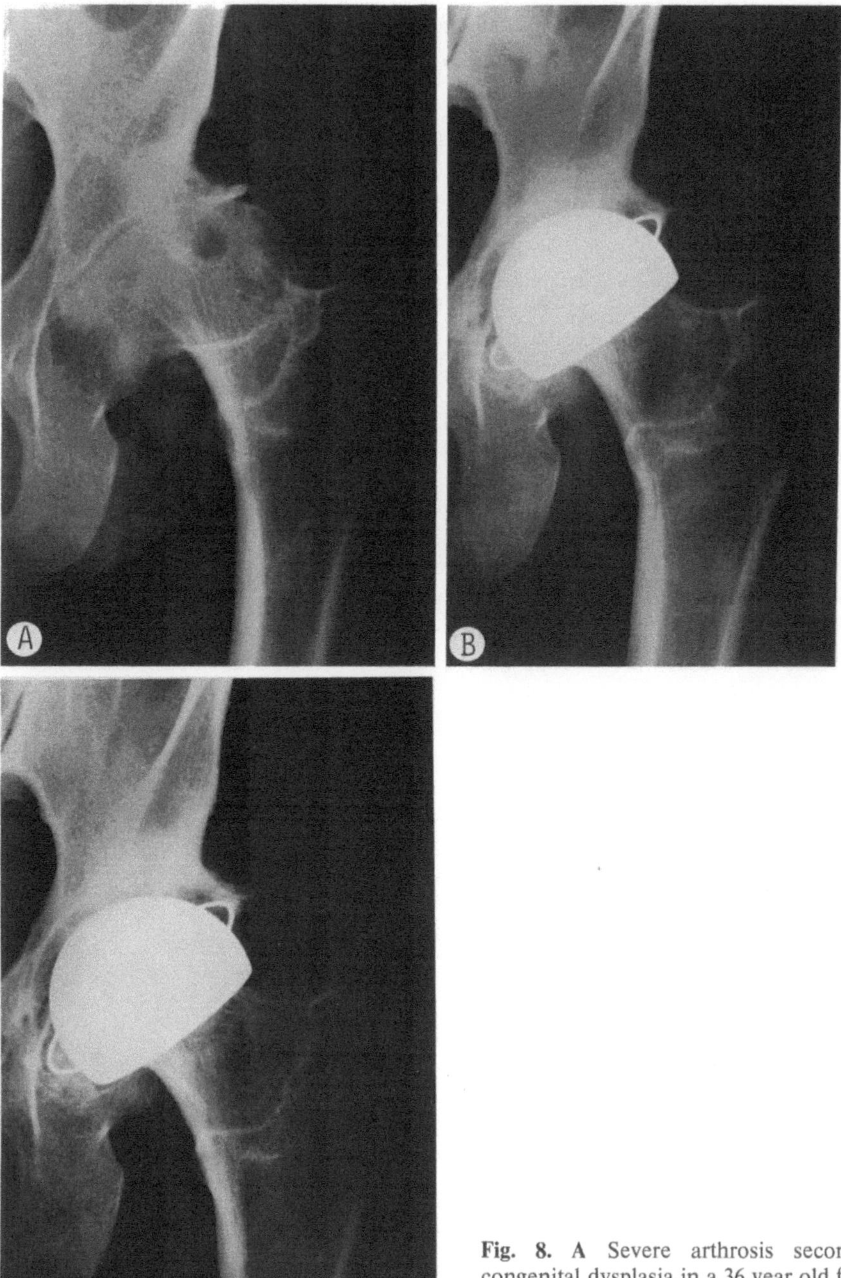

Fig. 8. A Severe arthrosis secondary to congenital dysplasia in a 36 year old female. **B** One year following resurfacing prosthesis. **C** Three years after operation

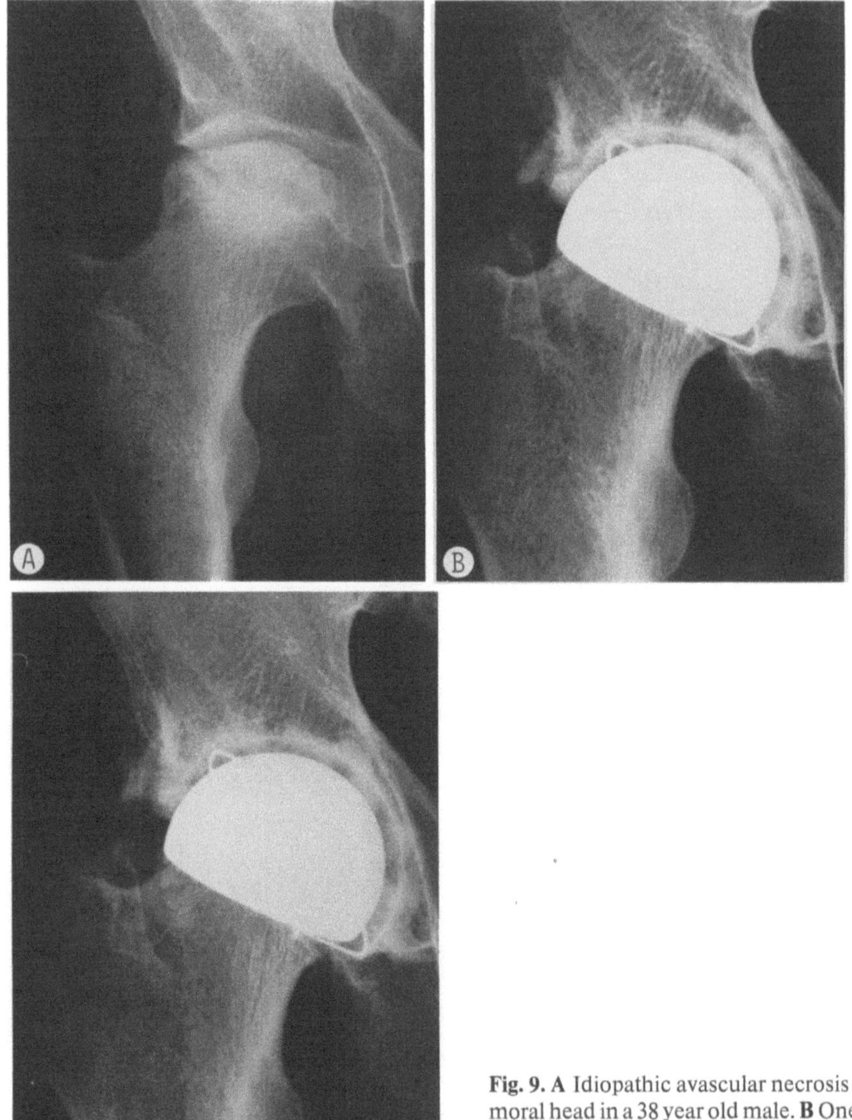

Fig. 9. A Idiopathic avascular necrosis of the femoral head in a 38 year old male. B One year following resurfacing prosthesis. C Three years after operation

are feasible, and therefore, (3) total hip replacement or arthrodesis are only reasonable alternatives.

Arthrodesis of the hip is understandably rarely accepted by the patient or physician and is generally contraindicated in bilateral hip disease. Total hip replacement has a restricted indication in the younger patient group. Resurfacing cannot be viewed as an alternative to total hip replacement. Thus, resurfacing is primarily indicated in the younger patient whose age is a relative contraindication to total hip replacement. Hip resurfacing is also a good alternative to arthrodesis since it restores painless function while retain-

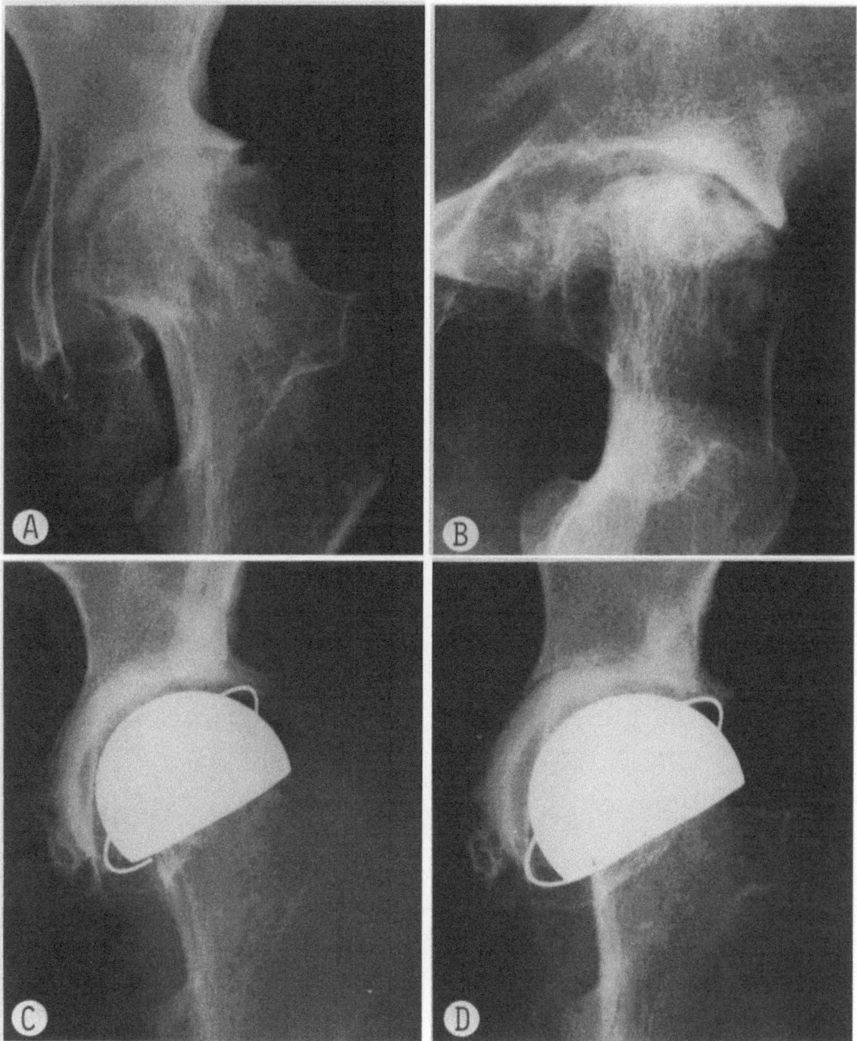

Fig. 10. A, B Partial avascular necrosis of the femoral head and painful partial fibrous ankylosis of the left hip in poor position in this 17 year old female. Status post slipped capital femoral epiphysis. **C** One year following surface replacement. **D** Three and a half years after operation

ing the original operative alternative should the resurfacing fail with time. Resurfacing offers a therapeutic alternative for younger patients who otherwise would be denied surgical treatment because they are too young for total hip replacement.

The use of the hip resurfacing procedure requires educating the patient. The patient's expectations and hopes of the prosthesis have to be carefully matched to his longevity, the urgency of the surgical procedure, other treatment alternatives, and to no treatment at all. Considering our relatively short experience, one cannot offer this type of joint replacement to someone with a life expectancy of thirty, forty, or fifty years and promise that it will last for his life time. Until long term followup is available, the resurfacing pros-

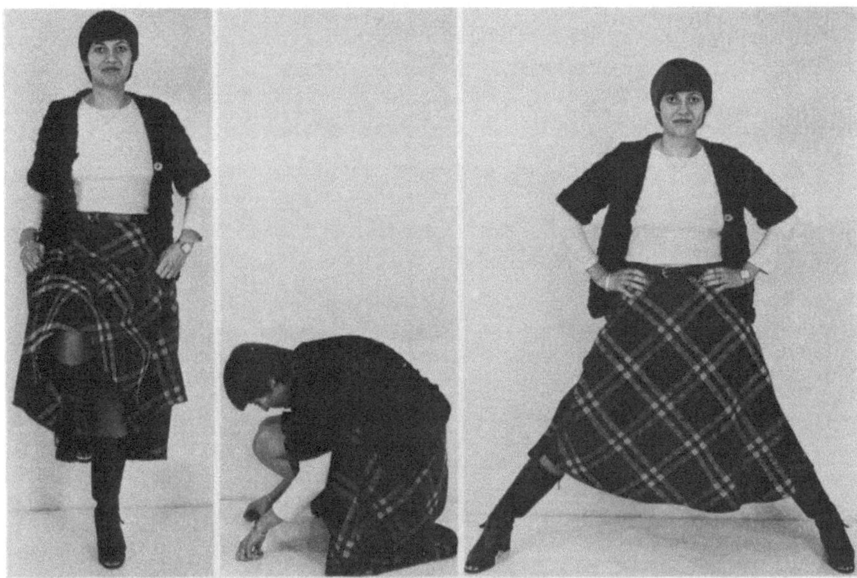

Fig. 11. Clinical photographs of the patient presented in Figure 10 taken three and a half years after resurfacing with the resurfacing endoprosthesis. She has essentially normal left hip function including a negative Trendelenburg test

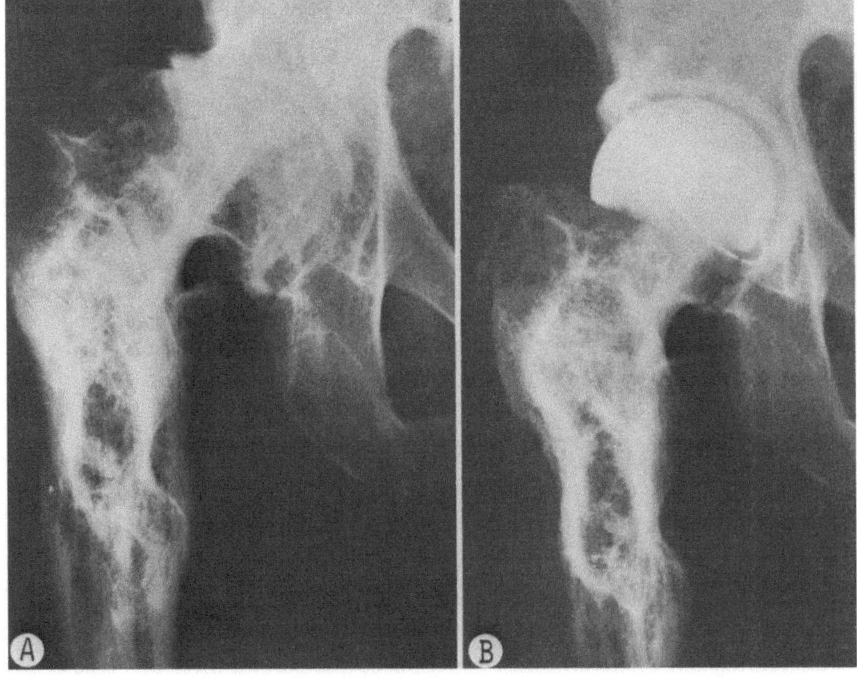

Fig. 12. Resurfacing prosthesis in severe coxarthrosis as a result of high velocity missile injury with proximal femur fracture and osteomyelitis

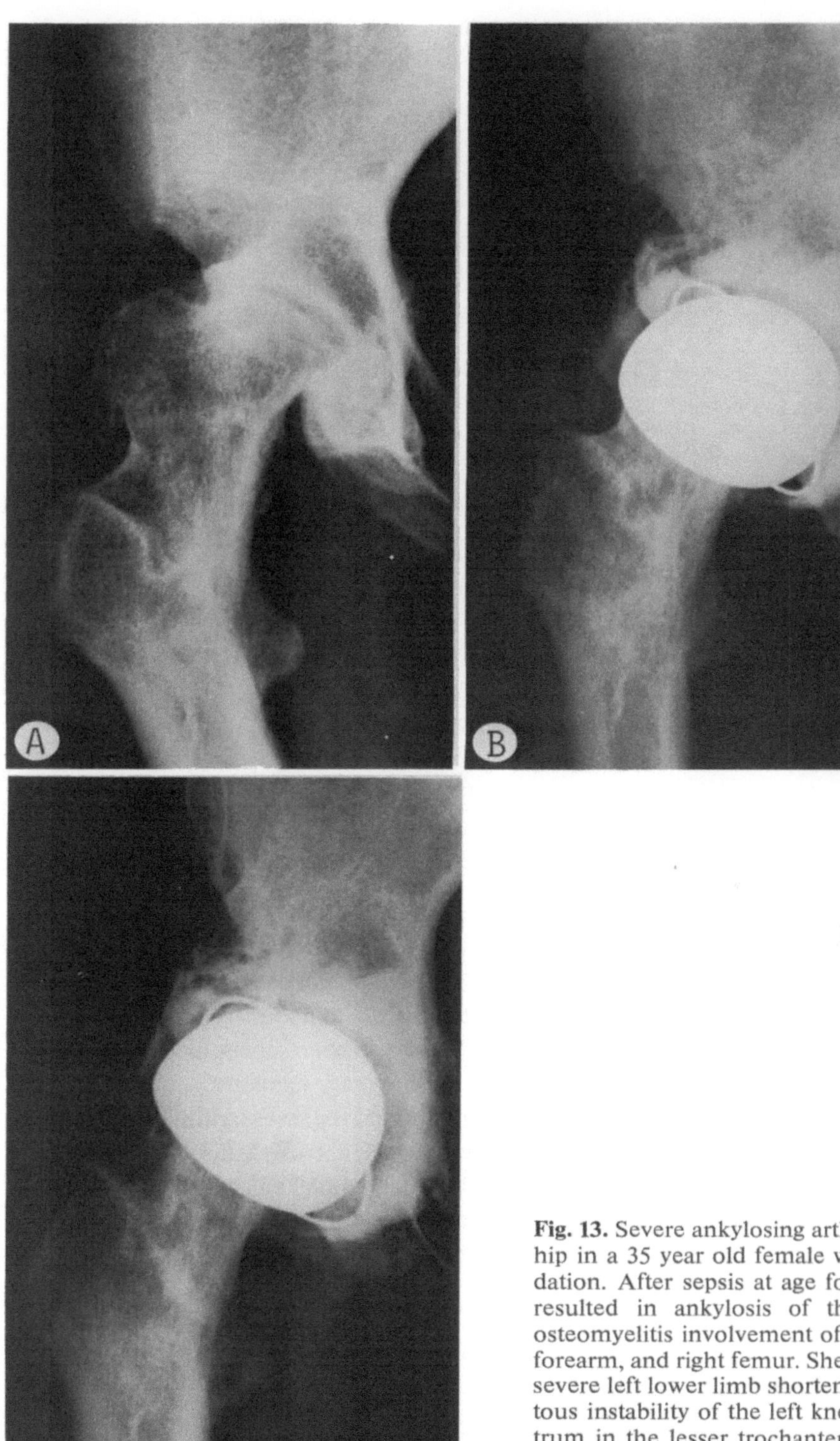

Fig. 13. Severe ankylosing arthrosis of the right hip in a 35 year old female with mental retardation. After sepsis at age four, osteomyelitis resulted in ankylosis of the left hip, and osteomyelitis involvement of both tibias, right forearm, and right femur. She also developed a severe left lower limb shortening and ligamentous instability of the left knee joint. (Sequestrum in the lesser trochanteric area). **B** Eight weeks following resurfacing of the right hip with bone grafting of the acetabular roof. **C** Four years following operation

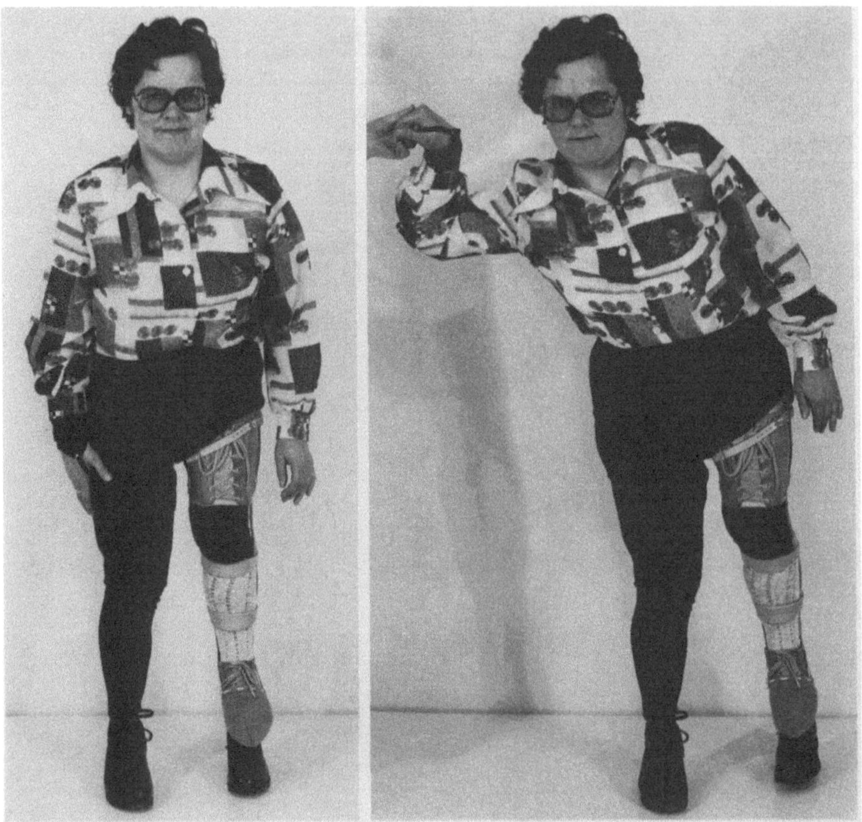

Fig. 14. Clinical photographs of the patient in figure 13 taken four years after resurfacing procedure of the right hip

thesis must be viewed as a temporizing measure. This does not decrease its value when done for the correct indications. After all, the principle of temporizing measures is not new to orthopaedics as evidenced by the use of classical joint preserving osteotomies for degenerative joint disease knowing they are only temporary solutions.

At this time, the best indications for resurfacing appear to be severe arthritis secondary to congenital dysplasia and advanced idiopathic avascular necrosis in the young patient. Painful stiff hips in poor position after slipped capital femoral epiphyses, and painful coxarthrosis in any age group secondary to septic arthritis or osteomyelitis are also indications for resurfacing (Figs. 8–14) since there are no alternative treatment methods availabe for these conditions.

Operative Technique

The operative technique can only be described briefly. The procedure is performed with the patient in the supine position on a flat radiolucent operating table. A 4 cm thick cushion is placed under the pelvis which has to be narrow enough to allow the lateral buttock to fall away posteriorly thus facilitating exposure. The joint is exposed through an anterior approach between the m. sartorius and m. tensor fasciae latae. The tensor fascia is incised longitudinally and the fibers of the tensor are carefully peeled away from its medial fascial covering, thus preserving the interspace between m. tensor and m. sartorius and eliminating the need for exposure of the lateral femoral cutaneous nerve. The interspace covered by the fascia containing the nerve is retracted medially and the tensor muscle is mobilized laterally. The abductor muscles are released from the outer surface of the ilium and lateral border of the iliac crest. To allow dislocation of the femoral head without force and undue muscle tension, soft tissue release has to be carried far enough posteriorly to release the entire gluteus medius and most of the gluteus minimus origins. If necessary, further release must be carried out during the dislocation maneuver. The subperiosteal elevation requires a very careful, delicate, and patient dissection in order to minimize postoperative scarring and heterotopic ossification of the hip muscle. In tight hips, especially those with flexion contractures, it may be necessary to extend the soft tissue dissection of the anterior third of the iliac crest onto the medial side mainly to reduce the tension on the sartorius and inguinal ligament.

The next step is to transect the origin of the straight head of the rectus femoris. The reflected head over the superior margin of the acetabulum is then resected: Capsular adhesions, so common in advanced coxarthrosis, have to be released. Frequently, the iliopsoas tendon has to be freed from its extensive scarred adhesions. With the hip slightly flexed to release the soft tissues, the iliopsoas may then be retracted with a periosteal elevator and a Hohmann retractor with a short, sharp spike driven into the superior pubic ramus 15 mm medial to the anterior acetabulum rim. This instrument allows medial retraction of the anterior soft tissue structures. The resection of the anterior and lateral portion of the capsule allows the dislocation of the femoral head. This is achieved by slowly flexing, abducting, and externally rotating the leg. During the dislocation maneuver it is necessary to frequently check the tension of the soft tissues. Further soft tissue release should be performed if indicated. From the moment of dislocation until the repositioning of the femoral head it is essential that the knee be flexed 90° in order to relax the sciatic nerve (Fig. 15).

The acetabulum and the femoral head are now prepared for implantation of the prosthetic cup. First, the osteophytic bone formation in the depths of the acetabulum is osteotomized with a gouge and removed. With the smallest reamer or large gouges, the acetabulum is deepened to the level of the fovea or inner cortex. Reamers of successively increasing diameters are then used to enlarge the acetabular diameter until a thickness of 4 to 5 mm remains on the anterior and posterior walls. An acetabular component of appropriate size is then selected.

The preservation of a 4–5 mm wall proved to be a good compromise because it preserves an acetabular wall that is sufficiently strong, but allows a prosthesis diameter large enough to conserve maximum bone stock on the femoral head.

During reaming of the acetabulum the sclerotic bone in the roof has to be preserved to guarantee a stable fixation of the implant. This bone is frequently the only segment capable of support. The reamed acetabulum is then notched throughout its circumference utilizing a 9 mm gouge. This is done to assure cement fixation. These notches have a width of 9 mm and a depth of 6–8 mm. Because of the elastic stress deformation of the

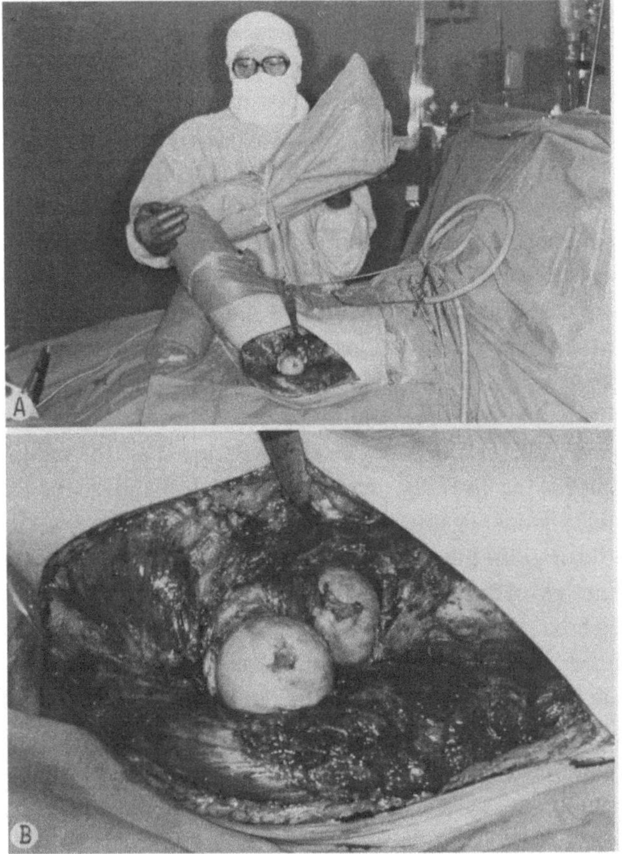

Fig. 15. A Positioning of the leg while the hip is dislocated. Note the 90° flexion of the knee and almost vertical position of the thigh. Note the cloth loop slung around the calf and tied to the Hohmann retractor to free the assistant's hands for support of the leg. A roll of sterile linen is also placed between the thighs to hold part of the weight of the leg. **B** Closeup of the operative site in (A). Note the excellent exposure of both the femoral head and acetabulum through the anterior approach

bony pelvis, it is advantageous to utilize ten to fifteen relatively small notches instead of the usual three 15 mm fixation holes. In addition, the multiple shallow notches preserve bone stock. This is important in the event that later removal and conversion to another treatment modality becomes necessary.

The polyethylene acetabular component is covered with a cone shaped layer of polymethylmethacrylate on its convex surface and then inserted into the prepared acetabulum utilizing the available instrumentation. First, several small rotary motions are made with the long handled inserter to insure better distribution of the cement of the bone surface. With this motion the excess cement is squeezed out of the acetabulum. Then the acetabular cup is firmly seated in its definitive position using the inserter. When it is removed the flange brings with it most of the excess cement. It is then exchanged for the pusher without a flange which is held with constant pressure until the cement hardens.

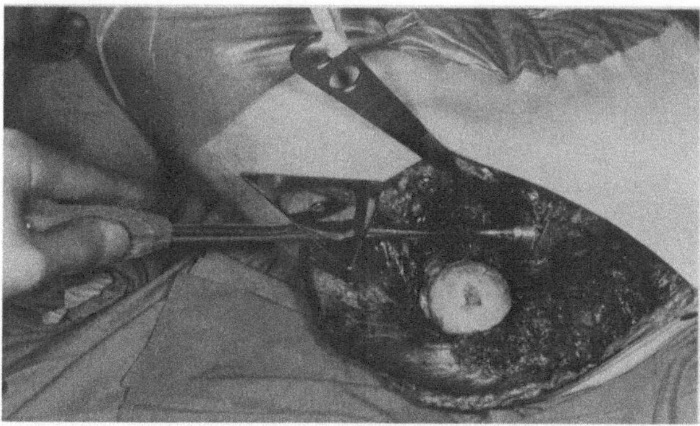

Fig. 16. The triangular alignment jig for the acetabular component can be attached to the positioning instrument. The jig is oriented parallel to the floor to create an anteversion of the acetabular component of 25°. The 45° inclination of the acetabular component is obtained by placing one leg of the alignment triangle parallel to the patients midline while the other limb is perpendicular to it

For fixation of the prosthetic cup one should strive for a 2 mm thick layer of cement. This has the advantage that only a small amount of cement, and more importantly, a small amount of monomer is implanted into the body. This thin layer of cement releases less heat of polymerization which causes no thermal tissue damage. An additional advantage is that the thin layer of cement is elastic and thus better follows the stress deformation of the bone and also that of the acetabular cup.

The best bone cement for obtaining a thin layer is one that remains pliable for several minutes and then hardens rapidly. In our hands the cement Sulfix-6 produced by Sulzer in Winterthur, Switzerland, has proven especially useful. This cement is stored at a temperature of +5 °C. Twenty-four hours prior to use, it is removed and placed at a constant room temperature of 22 °C. The polymerization of the mixed cement is timed with a stop watch. After vigorous mixing the semiliquid mixture is left undisturbed while entrapped air is allowed to escape. At eight minutes implantation can be started. After eleven minutes the cement has hardened. After more experience with the surgical technique has been gained, the starting time for mixing the cement can be determined while still preparing the acetabulum or the femoral head, so that no time need be lost while waiting for polymerization. The three minutes from beginning of implantation until the cement has hardened is a sufficiently short time that will not interrupt the rhythm of the procedure.

Training, experience, and skill are necessary to apply the appropriate amount of force and speed when pressing the implants with their cement linings into their prepared beds. Too slow an application will cause insufficient penetration of cement into the small irregularities of the bony surface. In addition, too much cement will remain interposed between the implant and the bone. Conversely, an implant seated too rapidly will gain contact with the supporting bone before the cement hardens. Even minimal movements during too rapid an insertion will cause complete cement voids at the interface, thereby creating less than optimal fixation. Unquestionably, these technical details contribute greatly to the life expectancy of the endoprosthesis.

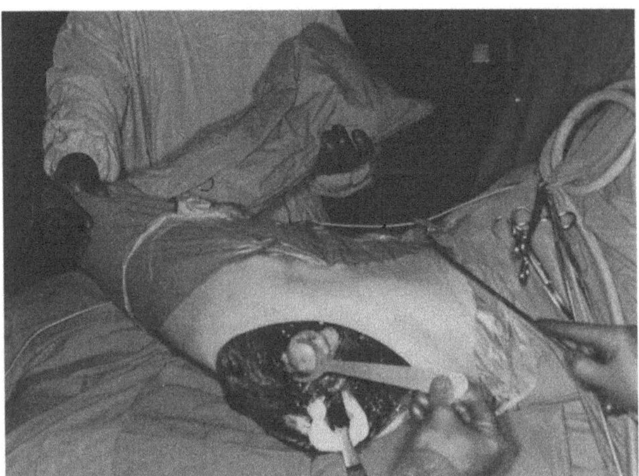

Fig. 17. Positioning of the leg during preparation of the femoral head

The most advantageous position for the acetabular component is 45° of abduction and 25° of flexion. To predetermine and later check this position, a very simple alignment jig has been developed. This instrument, which is basically an isosceles triangle, can be attached to the acetabular component applicator (Fig. 16). The acetabular component has been positioned correctly when the plane of the triangle is parallel to the floor and when one limb of the triangle is parallel to the body midline and the other perpendicular to it.

After insertion of the acetabular component, the limb is brought into a more relaxed position. The spiked Hohmann retractor is removed and replaced with a broad rake retractor. The thigh is allowed to rest on the opposite leg, the knee is flexed to 90° and the leg is held parallel to the floor (Fig. 17). The lateral soft tissues are retracted posteriorly utilizing a broad Hohmann type retractor placed underneath the greater trochanter. The femoral head and neck are now accessible from all sides.

The size of the femoral component to be used has been predetermined by the size of the already inserted acetabular component. The U-shaped femoral head gauge aids in determining the femoral head diameter which will accept the corresponding component and also help the surgeon to decide where redundant osteophytic bone has to be removed. Care must be taken not to violate the lateral and the dorsal structures of the femoral neck. Equally important is the preservation of the sclerotic bone in the cranial segment of the head which provides a stable base for fixation of the femoral cup. Another important detail is the placement of the implant in valgus as far laterally as possible (Fig. 1). As a rule of thumb, the femoral head has been correctly prepared when enough bone has been removed from the head to align the anterior and medial aspects of the head with those of the neck. The posterior neck has to be carefully protected because of the retinacular vessels in the area.

The excess bone is removed from the femoral head using an osteotome. The femoral head reamers are then used to obtain the final head shape starting with the largest reamer and finishing with the correct size to match the femoral component that was previously determined. The surface of the head is then prepared for cement fixation with multiple

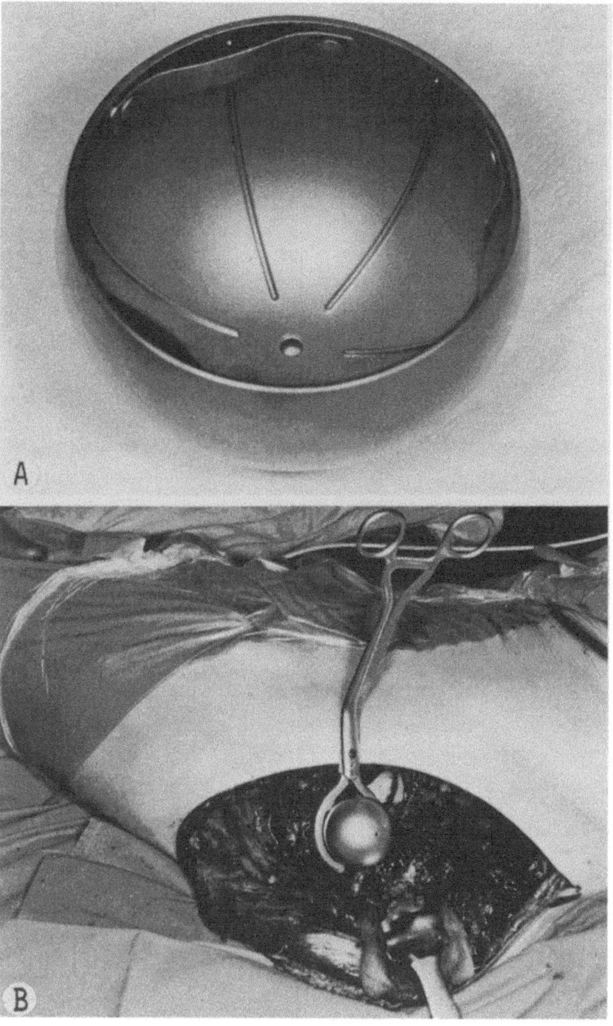

Fig. 18. A Trial femoral head component. This is held to the reamed femoral head by means of leaf springs along its inner margin. **B** After obtaining satisfactory position, the marking forceps are inserted parallel to the rim of the trial prosthesis. The trial prosthesis is then removed. The permanent femoral component is filled with cement and pushed over the head with the rim parallel to the marking forceps

shallow drill holes of 4.5 mm diameter and 4–5 mm in depth. The head is now ready to accept the implant.

In contrast to many other authors (Freeman, 1978; Amstutz, 1978), we emphasize the importance of preserving the retinacular vessels on the posterior aspect of the femoral neck. This is not to imply that severance of these vessels will inevitably lead to avascular necrosis of the head. However, after obliteration of the epiphysis, the femoral head has such a precarious blood supply that the contribution from the retinacular vessels has to be considered important (Hipp, 1962; Truetta and Harrison, 1953; Lanz and Wachsmuth,

1972). Their actual contribution to the blood supply of the head can be easily tested intraoperatively in most cases. After reaming, a sponge can be passed around the femoral neck for use as a tourniquet. The cancellous epiphyseal bony bleeding will decrease when the tourniquet is tightened by twisting the sponge and will resume when it has been released. Therefore, there is no reason to sacrifice these vessels, but rather one should preserve them to assure an optimal blood supply of the femoral head.

The femoral cup position is easily obtained using the femoral neck for orientation. An even more reliable control is possible by using the trial femoral prosthesis. This is a cup which has three leaf springs riveted along its inner rim to hold it on the prepared head and which permits a trial reduction (Fig. 18). Once reduced, the position of the trial cup can be accurately observed. With the leg in neutral position, the femoral cup should protrude from under the rim of the acetabular component by 15 mm. In neutral rotation and 15° abduction, the trial cup should completely disappear within the acetabulum as it also should in neutral rotation and 70° flexion with no abduction. Image intensification can also be used to verify the position. A single Kirschner wire is placed over the anterior superior iliac spine to provide orientation during this maneuver.

The femoral head is then redislocated and the marking forceps is placed around the neck parallel to the rim of the trial cup. This clamp has three teeth on its opposing semicircular surfaces which secure its position. The trial cup is then removed and the head is carefully cleaned one final time. The permanent prosthesis is lined with cement and slowly pressed over the head aligning the rim parallel to the marking forceps. Shortly prior to hardening, the excess cement is removed. A pointed plastic spatula is used to remove the cement from the central aperture.

After reduction of the femoral head, congruency of the prosthesis system is checked before reattachment of the musculature. The stability of the joint may be assessed by performing small rotary motions with the leg in neutral position. The range of internal rotation has to be checked. Sixty three percent of our patients had an external rotation contracture preoperatively. There is a risk of recurrence of this contracture if no attention is paid to the problem. There should be at least 40° of internal rotation obtained with ease prior to wound closure. If this is not obtained, a release of the posterior capsule is mandatory.

Wound closure is begun by reattaching the rectus femoris to the anterior inferior iliac spine. Four suction drainage tubes are placed at this time, two in the region of the joint and the other two along the iliac wing to prevent postoperative hematoma formation. The hip abductors are then reattached to the iliac crest with a running Dexon suture under little tension. The first two stitches of this suture are placed through bone immediately posterior to the anterior superior iliac spine. A fifth suction drainage tube is then placed subcutaneously and the subcutaneous tissue is then reapproximated. The skin is closed with a continuous subcuticular suture of monofilament nylon. Only then can the adherent plastic skin drape be removed and sterile dressings applied.

Preoperatively, the entire opposite limb and the leg on the operative side have been placed in elastic compression bandages. Postoperatively, the compression bandage is extended to include the operated joint and pelvis. The extremity is then placed in a foam rubber splint holding the leg in neutral rotation with slight flexion at the knee. Forty-eight hours postoperatively, the dressing and the suction drains are removed. Below knee compression bandages or elastic stockings are worn for an additional two weeks.

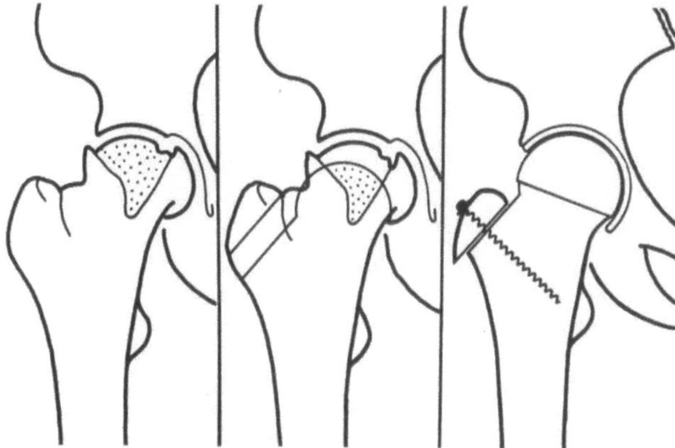

Fig. 19. Schematic diagram for femur preparation in a case of avascular necrosis. Bone is reamed from the femoral head until one half of the surface shows bleeding. The remaining necrotic tissue is then removed and the defect is packed with cancellous bone grafts. if reaming lads to excessive shortening of the femoral neck, transfer of the greater trochanter may be necessary

The resurfacing procedure may also be indicated in complex reconstructive procedures about the hip as in (1) remobilization of hip fusions, (2) destructive arthrosis secondary to dislocation, (3) severe acetabular destruction, and (4) severe proximal femoral destruction following previous surgery or congenital dislocation. For these cases, complex and rather involved modifications of the above described surgical technique are necessary. They can not be discussed here in detail.

However, we would like to point out the necessity of bone grafting which is encountered when dealing with the large areas of cystic degeneration, as well as arthrosis secondary to dysplasia and avascular necrosis. The necessary graft material can usually be obtained from osteophytes, or even better from ossifications in the depth of the acetabulum. Uti-

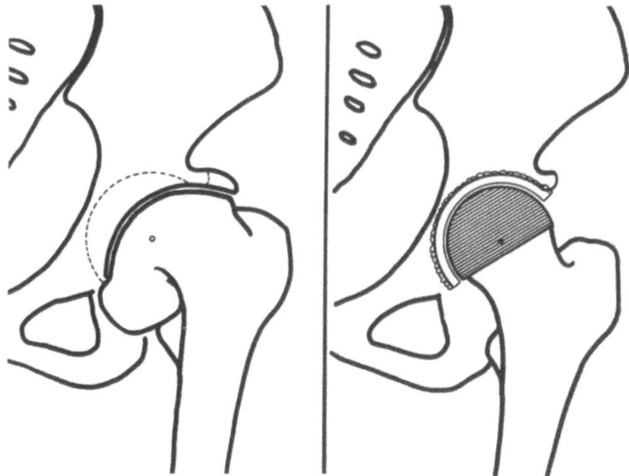

Fig. 20. Schematic diagram demonstrating the preservation of a superior osteophyte to allow coverage of the acetabular component in a dysplastic hip

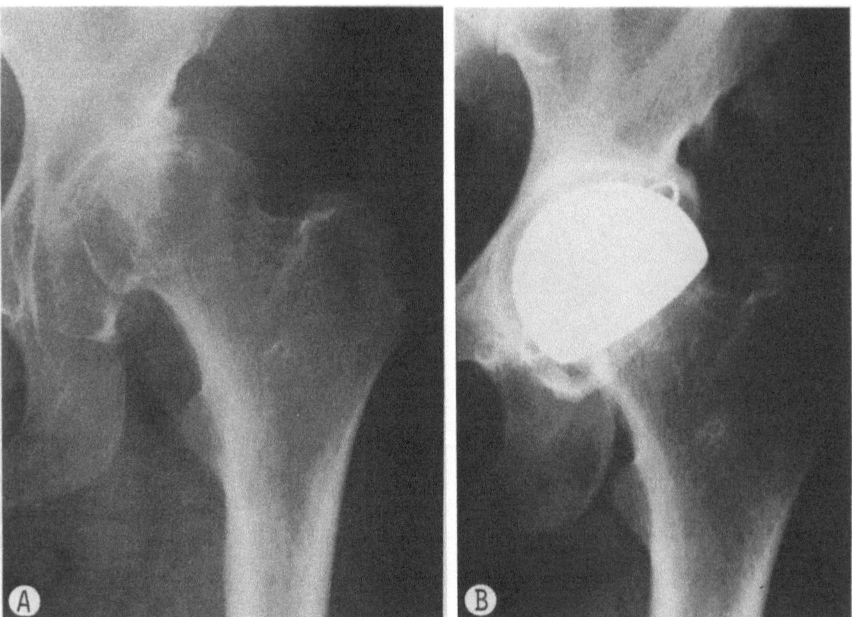

Fig. 21. A, B Radiograph of a 48 year old female with congenital dysplasia demonstrating the use of
the preserved superior osteophyte in covering the acetabular component

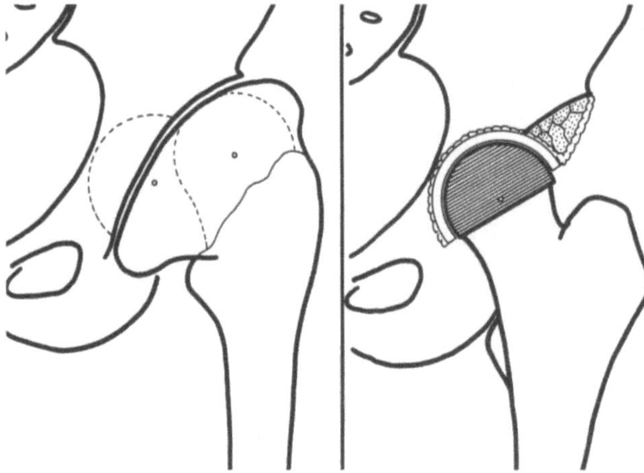

Fig. 22. Schematic diagram showing how coverage is obtained for the acetabular component with
cancellous bone grafts in coxarthosis with acetabular dysplasia. A flap of cement is used to hold the
grafts in position as is indicated in the drawing

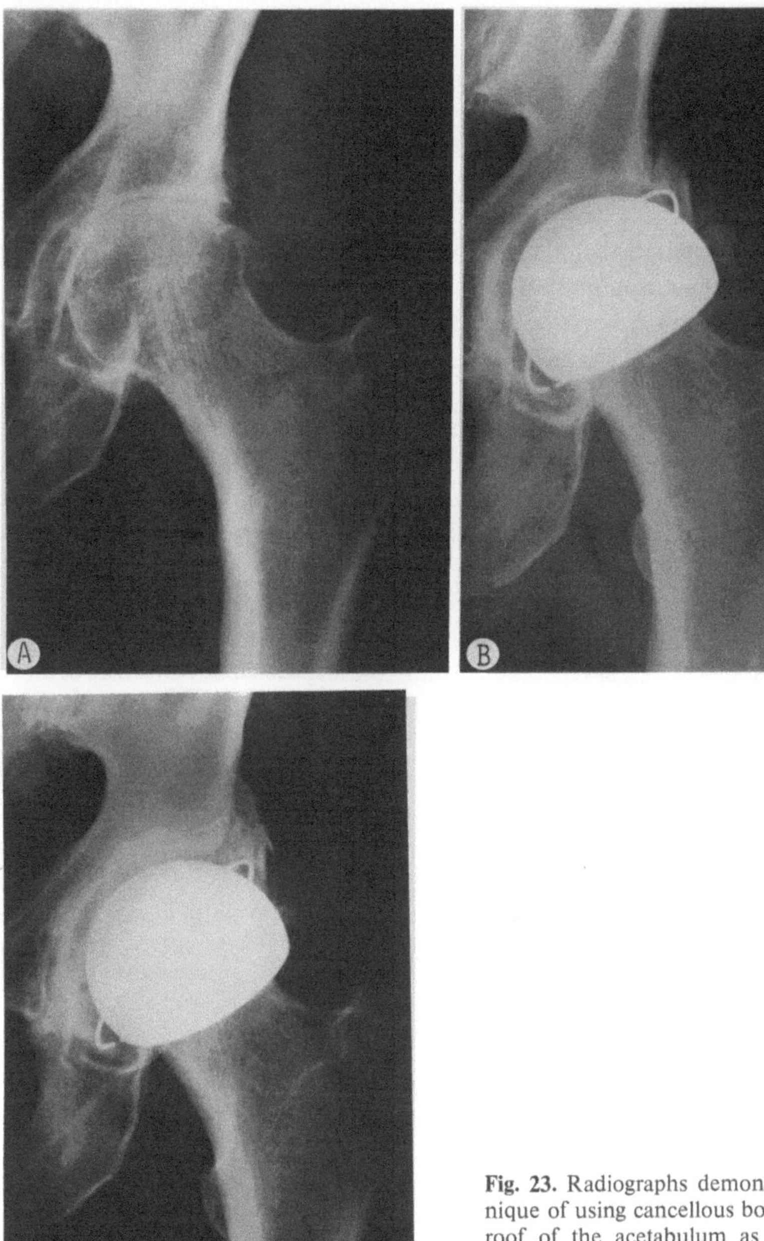

Fig. 23. Radiographs demonstrating the technique of using cancellous bone grafting at the roof of the acetabulum as in figure 22. **A** Coxarthrosis with an insufficient acetabulum in a 69 year old female. **B** Three weeks after resurfacing with bone grafting. **C** Two years after operation

lizing the anterior approach, the iliac crest is also available so that needed graft material may also be obtained from this location.

Arthrotic cysts of the femoral head and acetabulum which are exposed during reaming and which measure 8–10 mm in diameter require packing with cancellous bone after careful currettage. When defects which might influence the stability and the support of the prosthesis are grafted, it is important for the patient to remain on partial weight bearing using two crutches for a longer period of time. Grafting of these large arthrotic cysts is done with the idea that these grafts are incorporated within several weeks. They then become part of the femoral head while, if filled with polymethylmethacrylate this process would be prevented. After several years of clinical experience we have seen no tendency for the prosthesis to loosen following the use of bone grafts.

Another important indication for use of bone grafts to fill femoral head defects is in avascular necrosis of idiopathic and traumatic etiology. In these cases, more bone stock is removed from the femoral head than in cases of osteoarthritis. The bone is removed until approximately one half the reamed surface shows bleeding. The remaining necrotic bone is removed with a narrow gouge and the defect is packed with autologous cancellous bone grafts (Fig. 19). The femoral cup is inserted over this. If reaming of the bone stock results in significant shortening of the femoral neck, transposition of the greater trochanter distally and laterally may be indicated during this same procedure.

Acetabular dysplasia may also necessitate bone grafting when bony coverage of the superior or anterior aspects of the acetabular component is inadequate because of hypoplasia of the acetabulum. The easiest solution for this problem is provided where a cup-shaped osteophyte has been formed as a result of the arthritis. This osteophyte can be utilized to provide coverage for the prosthesis (Figs. 20 and 21). If such an osteophyte is not present, one has to judge after acetabular reaming if there is sufficient depth of the acetabulum to provide adequate stability for the implant. In those cases in which stability is sufficient but coverage is inadequate, the outer aspect of the ilium directly above the

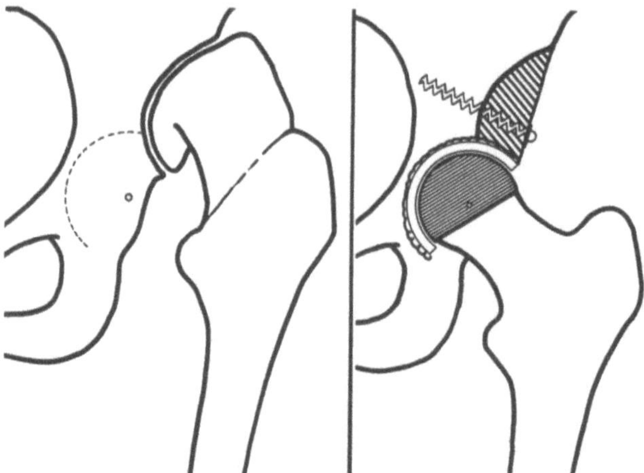

Fig. 24. Schematic diagrams of coxarthrosis secondary to dislocation demonstrating the reconstruction of the acetabular roof by a corticocancellous bone graft fixed with screws

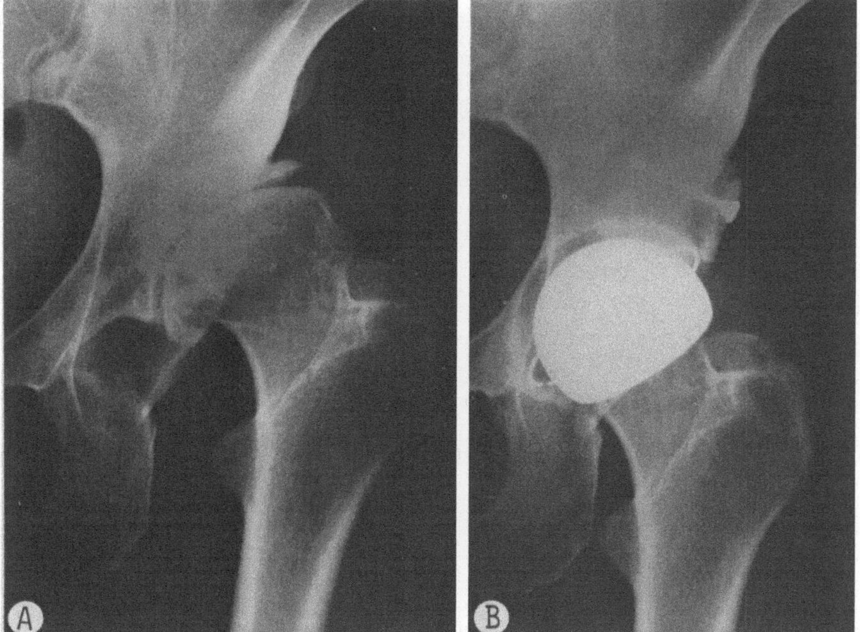

Fig. 25. A, B Radiographs of a 43 year old female with coxarthrosis secondary to dislocation. Acetabular reconstruction using a corticocancellous graft held with a single screw

acetabular rim is decorticated and perforated with multiple small holes. When inserting the acetabular component the cement escaping superiorly is preserved as a continuous flap. Cancellous bone grafts are placed above the protruding rim of the acetabular component and then the flap of cement is folded around the graft. This is held in place until the cement hardens (Figs. 22 and 23). The very thin cement flap is only expected to provide stability for the graft until it has fused to the ilium. It does not have the purpose of providing mechanical support for the implant.

If the reamed acetabulum does not appear deep enough to provide adequate stability for the firm seating of the component, the acetabular rim has to be extended with the use of a bone graft. This is accomplished by fixing a curved corticocancellous graft to the supraacetabular area with screws. This graft, in contrast to the multiple cancellous bone chips, does provide immediate support by virtue of its screw fixation (Figs. 24 and 25).

Postoperative Management

The preoperative and postoperative treatment requires the same careful attention to detail as does the operative procedure. Normally the patient is admitted three or four days prior to surgery. During this time a number of important diagnostic and therapeutic measures are performed. At the same time the patient can adjust to hospital routine while being protected from everyday stresses. The anesthesiologist has the opportunity to

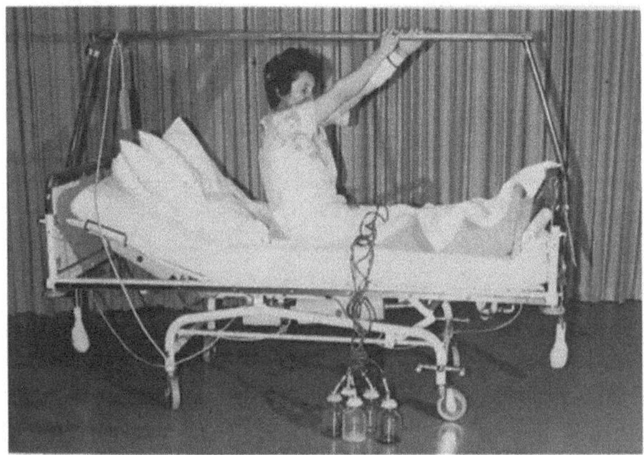

Fig. 26. Sitting up exercises are begun on the first postoperative day (Electric orthopaedic hospital bed).

arrange for auto-transfusion. The usual routine involves the removal of 1500 ml of blood three days prior to surgery. This volume is replaced with plasma expanders at that time. Thus, surgery is performed in a state of relative hemodilution and auto-transfusions are begun during surgery and continued postoperatively if needed. This eliminates the risk inherent in a donor transfusion.

Physical therapy is also initiated preoperatively. Specifically the patient is instructed in breathing exercises, isometric muscle training and the use of Loftstrand crutches. Using a bathroom scale, the patient is taught to partially weight bear on his involved extremity. Eventually, sitting-up exercises are practiced. The hospital bed utilized is equipped with a longitudinal overhead bar which allows the patient to pull himself into a sitting position while providing good hand grasps at each level of inclination. This and the fact that the bed is automatically adjustable allows the patient to become significantly independent very early in the postoperative phase.

Deep breathing and sitting up exercises are begun on the first postoperative day. Three times a day the patient gets up to stand at the bedside in an upright position. Ambulation is begun on the third postoperative day in the room and the patient is allowed to sit up at the bedside for short periods. Ambulation is extended throughout the ward on postoperative day five and isometric tightening exercises of the gluteal muscles are begun in the prone position. On the fifteenth postoperative day active abduction exercises against gravity in the lateral decubitus position are started. Also at this time, partial weight bearing using only one forearm crutch in the opposite hand is begun and the patients are taught stair climbing. Most patients are discharged on the twenty-first postoperative day and are instructed to continue their exercises at home for five more weeks, a total of two months. Active flexion exercises are not allowed.

Radiographs are obtained immediately postoperatively, at three weeks when discharged, and then at three months. Most patients are allowed to discard their remaining forearm crutch at two to three months. However, those who have undergone bone grafting are usually maintained partial weight bearing on crutches for up to six months. Further radiographs are obtained at six months and then at yearly intervals unless problems arise.

Range of motion exercises have not been proven to be beneficial as a form of physical therapy postoperatively. They seem to cause an increase in periarticular heterotopic bone formation rather than the expected increase in mobility for which they are often instituted. We have observed an optimal recovery of joint mobility in those patients who were allowed to find their own level of functional activity as long as it did not cause them any pain.

Discussion of Results

Hip resurfacing has a long history. Probably the earliest attempts to resurface the hip date back to the beginning of this century (Pupovac, Lexer) when biologic material was used in interpositional arthroplasties. In 1939, Smith-Peterson described the use of a hemispherical metal cup in his interpositional arthroplasty of the hip which gained wide acceptance. Smith-Peterson had hoped, as did Pauwels several years later, to produce a fibrocartilaginous lining as the result of motion of bone against the smooth metallic surface. Gerard has modified this concept by interposing two concentric cups which allowed motion between themselves as well as between the cups and the bone.

Bone resorption has been found to occur wherever bone comes into contact with movable implants, whether constructed of metal or plastic. This finding has inspired a number of authors to use polymethylmethacrylate for the fixation of the components used in hip joint surface replacement. Paltrinieri and Trentani, as well as Furuya, used metal cups as a covering for the femoral head articular surface. These had a flange-type collar which extended down onto the femoral neck and thus enclosed a relatively large amount of bone stock. Freeman has worked with a number of modifications over the last several years and has also developed a cemented double cup endoprosthetic replacement for the hip. His technique reduces the femoral head to a cylindrical stump which is inserted into the corresponding cylindrical cavity of the femoral cup. Further modifications have been described recently by Amstutz, Eicher and Capello, Nishio, Tanaky, and Salzer, et. al.

The surface replacement endoprosthesis system which we developed is distinguished by its thin walls for bone conservation. It extends over the area of the natural articular surface minimizing the amount of bone encased by the foreign body. The results of resur-

Table 1. Postoperative followup on 659 resurfacing procedures

Follow up time	
> 4 years	25 hips
> 3 years	46 hips
> 2 years	141 hips
> 1 year	288 hips
< 1 year	159 hips
total	659 hips

Table 2. Average pre- and postoperative range of motion. (Data obtained from follow up examinations of 426 hips one year prior to this publication)

Range of Motion	Preop	Postop
Flexion-Extension	60.3°	76.4°
Abduction-Adduction	21.8°	44.2°
Rotation	14.6°	39.7°

facing are very promising to date. It fills an important gap in the therapeutic armamentarium primarily when dealing with severely disabled younger patients. Reliable statistical data is not yet available due to the short followup time. The longest followup is more than five years and only a few procedures were performed during the first two years (Table 1). This means that the majority of the patients have been followed for less than three years. This observation time is too short to rely on for help in complex decision making in patients, the majority of whom usually have long life expectancy. This fact in itself demands a critical and conservative approach in the selection of patients for resurfacing only when operative treatment is inevitable, and, secondary to the severity of the symptoms only when total prosthetic replacement or arthrodesis are the only remaining alternatives.

As is evident from the preoperative restriction of motion (Table 2), the resurfacing prosthesis was used only in patients with advanced disease. Those with a better range of motion were treated with joint conserving osteotomies. The increase in the range of motion postoperatively was most significant in rotation and least apparent in flexion/extension. In most patients a slow spontaneous improvement in range of motion is noted over the first two years postoperatively. In general, the patient with good preoperative range of motion has better mobility postoperatively. To average the values of range of motion as was done in table 2 can be deceiving since it does not demonstrate the varying results with different forms of arthrosis. Patients with arthrosis secondary to hip dysplasia gain a great deal of mobility. Patients with tight hips who have extensive acetabular osteophyte formation and circumferentially protruding osteophytes will gain little mobility or may actually lose range of motion. These problems can only be related to different forms of arthrosis through future followup examinations.

An important problem in resurfacing, as in any other procedure on the hip joint, is periarticular ossification. In 4% we have noted severe ossification with marked limitation of motion. In 15% of joints that were resurfaced, a moderate amount of heterotopic bone formation was found but its effect on the functional limitation of the patients could not be quantified. Restriction of motion and extent of heterotopic bone formation are by no means closely related. There are marked restrictions in range of motion without ossification and there are cases of extensive heterotopic bone formation without significant limitation of function.

Heterotopic bone formation is probably a phenomenon related to the patient's constitution. The surgical wound is only one of the important etiological factors. In arthrosis secondary to dysplasia heterotopic ossification is rare. The appearance of heterotopic bone is common if the medial acetabulum has a large osteophyte and an inferior collar of osteophytes. Alcoholic patients also tend to develop extensive soft tissue ossification.

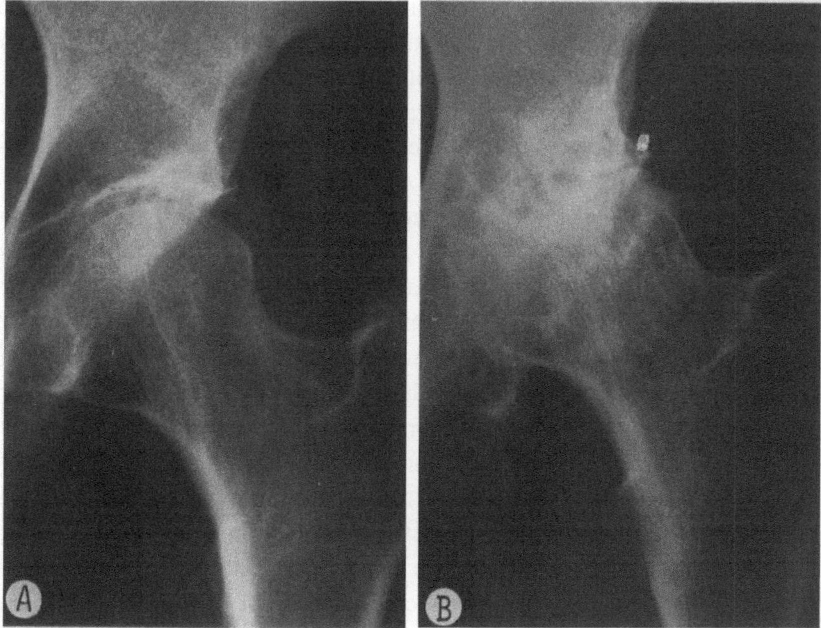

Fig. 27. Inflammatory coxarthrosis with progressive reactive osteolysis in a 72 year old female. **A** At age 72 when she first developed symptoms. **B** One year later with severe destruction of the hip joint

Patients susceptible to periarticular ossification can be recognized during pre- and post-operative examination of their locomotor system by their inability to relax their musculature. Accordingly, we have used a peripheral muscle relaxant, methylcarbamol[2] for the first three weeks postoperatively in all patients. We have noted a decrease in ossification with this regime but are still unable to verify this with statistical data.

The most important problem in hip resurfacing is still the loosening of the implant. It is obvious that the longevity of the prosthetic implant is related to the quality of the underlying bone. Therefore it is no surprise to find the majority of prosthetic loosenings in patients with poor bone stock. This occurs most often in inflammatory arthrosis with rapidly progressive resorption of the bone (Fig. 27). In contrast to this, in idiopathic avascular necrosis where we expected a high incidence of loosening, we have, to our surprise, found no case of loosening to date.

According to our present knowledge, we recognise inflammatory arthrosis with reactive atrophy and bone resorption as a relative contraindication for resurfacing. The therapeutic dilemma in dealing with this disease is difficult because the severe pain forces the physician to use surgical treatment and yet the poor bone stock makes total hip replacement equally unacceptable as a therapeutic alternative. For want of a better solution, we are currently approaching the problem by removing all of the atropic, hyperemic subchondral bone. Experience with this method is too limited to allow definite conclusions

---

[2] *Robaxin.* A. H. Robbins Company, Richmond, Virginia.

to be drawn. It must be emphasized that inflammatory hip disease with reactive bone resorption presents an increased risk for loosening of the components. Therefore, resurfacing with the double cup endoprosthesis is not indicated in these patients as long as any alternative therapeutic modalities remain available. However the increased risk of prosthetic loosening in a patient who requires an alloplastic joint replacement may influence the surgeon to make a decision in favor of resurfacing. This is because resurfacing offers the advantage that removal of loosened components is much easier than after total hip replacement.

Loose resurfacing components can be replaced immediately if the remaining bone stock is sufficient. If the bone stock in the femoral head is inadequate the resurfacing endoprosthesis can be converted to a total hip replacement. Even simple removal of the components is a very acceptable salvage procedure providing there was a good indication for the original resurfacing procedure. A lateral and distal transfer of the greater trochanter is performed at the same time as the components are removed, and the patient is kept on partial weight bearing. These patients have much more hip stability than those who have undergone removal of a total hip prosthesis. We are currently following several patients after this component removal and note that they are relatively pain free and have good mobility. Radiographic evidence of an increasing radiolucency along the joint surface is observed in these patients which represents the formation of a new fibrocartilaginous joint surface.

Replacement or removal of the components has occurred in 18 cases to date. Twelve of these were in patients whose resurfacing had been done for symptoms secondary to inflammatory arthrosis. These cases developed their loosening in the second and third years after resurfacing and none occurred in the first postoperative year. Of the remaining four cases one occurred in a patient with atrophic bone following multiple osteotomies which were performed for the realignment of a dysplatic hip. In the second, radiographs showed a thin-walled cyst of 1.5 cm diameter in the superolateral segment of the femoral head. The femoral endoprosthetic component, which had been implanted in an excessive varus position, fractured the lateral cortex of the femoral neck under the excessive stress of the patient's heavy physical labor. The third patient required removal of the components because of a late infection occurring one year after surgery. These components were found to be very well fixed to the underlying bone with no signs of loosening. The last of these cases was a patient who developed a hip infection a few days after septic tonsillitis. We suspect hematogenous inoculation since this patient was one year post resurfacing and had been symptom free prior to that time. Under systemic antibiotic coverage, revision of the hip joint was performed. The acetabular component was removed because granulation tissue was found along the exposed bone-cement interface although it was not demonstrated to be loose. A new acetabular component was inserted utilizing Gentamycin impregnated cement. Primary wound healing occurred and there were no postoperative problems. The patient has become asymptomatic since discharge. However his followup time since revision is only six months.

Two patients have sustained subcapital fractures of the femoral neck and account for the last two cases of revision. One of these complications occurred in a 36 year old male with rheumatoid spondylitis who had severe inflammatory, destructive changes of one hip. He sustained a femoral neck fracture on the tenth postoperative day. On reexploration, a large cyst was found at the head-neck junction area which involved the entire diameter of the neck. This cyst was not visible on preoperative roentgenograms. A pathological fracture had occurred through the thin wall of the cyst. After transfer of the greater trochanter, a new femoral prosthesis was placed over the femoral neck.

The other case which was complicated by a subcapital neck fracture occurred in a patient where the head had been surrounded by a large osteophyte. Removal of this osteophyte left an area of atrophic bone in the subcapital region which fractured through apparent overuse. This patient was converted to a total hip prosthesis (Fig. 7).

Other problems and complication are of relative insignificance. For example, in over 600 procedures there has been only one case of pulmonary embolism detected on a clinical basis but fibrinogen scans were not utilized. This patient recovered without sequelae. Anticoagulants and antiplatelet drugs were not used.

The patients who underwent resurfacings present a broad spectrum of disease and careful long term followup will be necessary before a reliable analysis of the indications and results can be obtained.

The most gratifying results were obtained in severely incapacitated young patients. In this group, there is no real alternative because of the severity of the findings and the age of the patient. On the other hand, they have good bone stock for stable fixation of the implants. Other cases particularly suited for resurfacing include degenerative arthrosis with sclerotic joint margins, avascular necrosis of the femoral head, fibrous partial ankylosis following slipped capital femoral epiphysis, and degenerative arthrosis following osteomyelitis of the hip area or septic arthrosis of the hip.

Summary

After five years of followup, the resurfacing procedure of the hip joint has proven to be a valuable addition to our therapeutic armamentarium. Indications for this procedure, especially in younger patients, are present only when pain and disability demand surgical treatment, when joint preserving osteotomies can not be expected to be effective, or when total hip prosthesis or arthrodesis remain as the only alternatives. The longevity of the prosthesis is largely dependent upon the quality of the bone stock. Inflammatory arthrosis with bone atrophy and progressive reactive bone resorption presents an increased risk for prosthetic loosening.

Acknowledgement: The author gratefully acknowledges Winfried M. Berger, M.D., LTC MC USA, Altdorf bei Nürnberg, West Germany and Roger W. Hood, M.D., Boston, Massachusetts for translating this paper.

References

Amstutz HC, Graff-Radford A, Gruen ThA, Clarke JC (1978) Tharies surface replacements: A review of the first 100 cases. Clin Orthop 134:87
Capello W, Ireland PhH, Trammell TR, Eicher P (1978) Conservative total hip arthroplasty: A procedure to conserve bone stock – Part I and Part II. Clin Orthop 134:59

Freeman MAR (1978) Some antomical and mechanical considerations relevant to the surface
    replacement of the femoral head. Clin Orthop 134:19
Freeman MAR, Cameron HU, Brown GC (1978) Cemented double cup arthroplasty of the hip:
    A 5 year experience with the ICLH prosthesis. Clin Orthop 134:45
Furuya K, Tschuchiya M, Kawachi S (1978) Socket-cup arthroplasty. Clin Orthop 134:41
Gérard Y, Ségal Ph, Nedoucha JS (1974) L'arthroplastie de la hanche par cupules couplées. Rev
    Chir orthop (Suppl. II) 60:281
Gérard Y (1978) Hip arthroplasty by matching cups. Clin Ortop 134:25
Grünert A, Ritter G (1973) Experimentelle Untersuchungen zum Problem der Verankerung von
    Hüftendoprothesen. Arch orthop Unf Chir 77:149
Hipp E (1962) Die Gefäße des Hüftkopfes. Enke, Stuttgart
Lanz J, Wachsmuth W (1972) Praktische Anatomie. Bein und Statik, Bd. 1/IV. Springer Berlin
Lexer E (1916) Die Verwertung der freien Fettgewebsverpflanzung zur Wiederherstellung und
    Erhaltung der Gelenkbeweglichkeit. Dtsch Z Chir 135:389
Nishio A, Eguchi M, Kaibara N (1978) Socket and cup surface replacement of the hip. Clin Orthop
    134, 53
Pauwels F (1960) Eine neue Theorie über den Einfluß mechanischer Reize auf die Differen-
    zierung der Stützgewebe. Z Anat Entwickl Gesch 121:478
Pupovac F (1912) Zur Verwendung ungestielter Lappen aus der Fascia lata bei der Mobilisierung
    ankylosierter Gelenke. Wein klin Wochenschr 521
Ritter G, Grümert A, Schweikert CH (1973) Biomechanische Ursachen von Lockerung und
    Bruch der Hüftendoprothesen. Arch orthop Unf Chir 77:154
Salzer M, Kmahr K, Locke H, Stärk N (1978) Cement-free bioceramic double-cup endoprosthesis
    of the hip-joint. Clin Orthop 134:80
Smith-Peterson MN (1939) Arthroplasty of the hip. A new method. J Bone Joint Surg 21:269
Tanaka S (1978) Surface replacement of the hip joint. Clin Orthop 134:75
Trentani C, Vaccarino F (1978) The Paltrinieri-Trentani hip joint resurface arthroplasty. Clin
    Orthop 134:36
Trueta J, Harrison MHM (1953) The normal vascular anatomy of the femoral head in adult man.
    J Bone Joint Surg 35B:442
Wagner H (1968) Ätiologie, Pathogenese, Klinik und Therapie der idiopathischen Hüftkopfne-
    krose. Verth Dtsch Orthop Ges 54:224
Wagner H (1972) Möglichkeiten und klinische Erfahrungen mit der Knorpeltransplantation. Z
    Orthop 110:705
Wagner H (1975) Der alloplastische Gelenkflächenersatz am Hüftgelenk. Arch Orthop Unf Chir
    82:101
Wagner H (1978) Surface replacement arthoplasty of the hip. Clin Orthop 134:102

Translation from the German: Wagner H (1979) Die Schalenprothese des Hüftgelenkes – Ober-
flächen-Ersatz als Gelenkerhaltung. In: Der Orthopäde 8:276–295 © Springer Verlag 1979

Long Term Results of Chiari Pelvic Osteotomies

A. Schreiber

Since 1962 we performed in our hospital over 500 pelvic osteotomies as first presented by Chiari in 1956. Winkler and Weber reported in 1977 on the results of 203 cases; Ieda and Winkler published the results of 55 operations performed on pre-school age children with an average observation period of 11.5 years in 1979. We presented the outcome of 51 osteotomies carried out 10–19 years ago on patients who had reached bony maturity at the SOFCOT convention in Paris in 1975. Discussion at that time dealt with the influence of Chiari pelvic osteotomy on coxarthrosis.

It is unnecessary therefore to repeat the basic concepts of this procedure, but we have to point out that we have changed our opinion concerning its indications. Until 1972, Chiari pelvic osteotomy was performed mainly in cases of acetabular dysplasia. After this date, we used nearly exclusively the Salter pelvic osteotomy or an acetabuloplasty for children under the age of 6. Exceptions were cases with a very small and steep acetabular roof. We began to employ the Chiari pelvic osteotomy for an increasing number of older patients and finally for patients with an established coxarthrosis. This report deals mainly with the last mentioned cases. We will not repeat previously published statistics.

The goal of the operation is to create a large and congruent coverage for the femoral head. Medialisation of the center of joint motion changes effectiveness and the lever arm of the pelvitrochanteric musculature. It is impossible to achieve primary congruence of the joint surfaces even by employing an arc-shaped osteotomy. Such an attempt makes the operation more difficult and medialisation is harder to achieve. It is better to make a level cut with a slight ascent in a dorsolateral to a ventromedial direction. In this simple manner, one achieves very good displacement. The ventral gap between the femoral head (capsule) and the osteotomy site can be filled with a bone graft. The graft is obtained from the iliac crest or from the intertrochanteric area in cases of a simultaneous intertrochanteric osteotomy.

In about one half of our patients we performed an intertrochanteric osteotomy, either simultaneously with the pelvic osteotomy or at a second stage. In such situations, it is important to obtain functional X-rays prior to the operation. One is tempted to consider a varus osteotomy in the presence of a coxarthrosis combined with subluxation, but valgus osteotomy combined with a Chiari pelvic osteotomy will provide a much larger weight bearing joint surface for the misshapen femoral head in spite of the presence of subluxation. It is surprising to observe the development of congruent joint surfaces, even after cessation of bone growth. This change is caused by functional adaptation of the acetabular roof.

Clinical Results

In considering only those patients in whom a more or less pronounced arthrosis was present at the time of surgery and who had been followed postoperatively for a period of more than 10 years, clinical results graded according to the Merle d'Aubigné point system are at first sight disappointing. Only slightly more than one half can be graded as good. Merle d'Aubigné's system makes too much allowance for rotation, which becomes markedly limited after a Chiari pelvic osteotomy. Also the diminution of pain is not properly con-

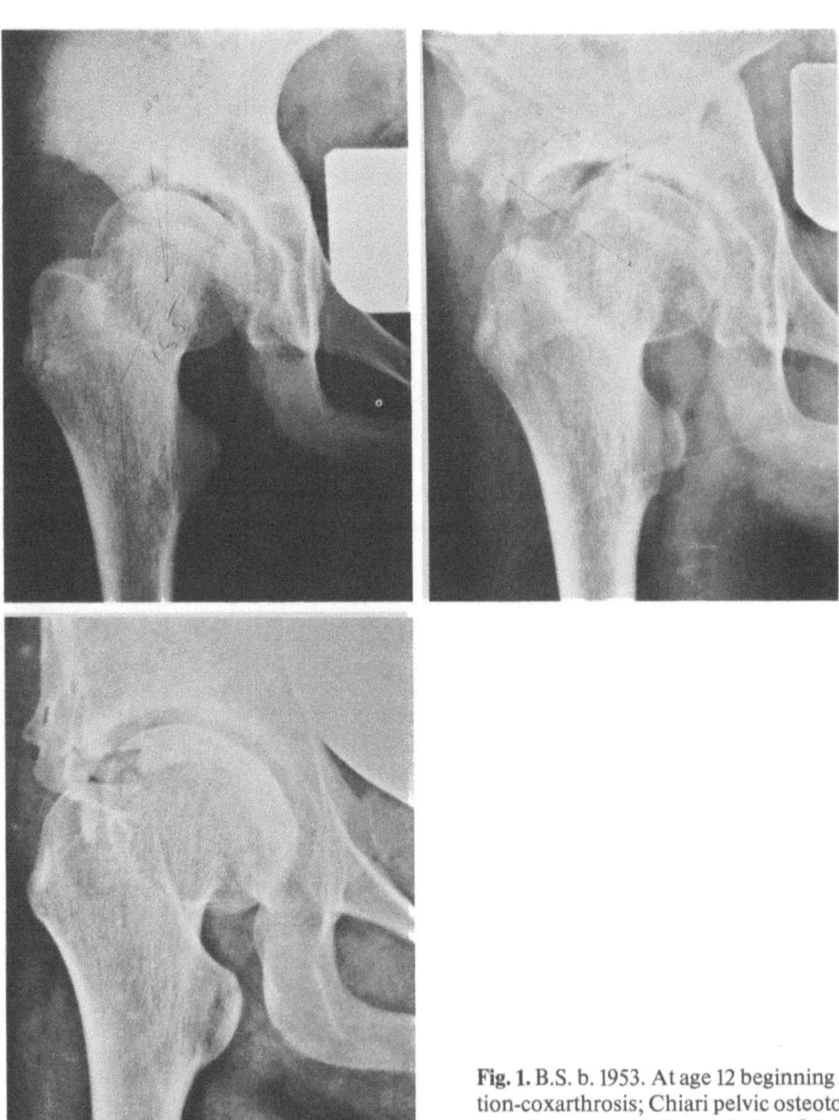

Fig. 1. B.S. b. 1953. At age 12 beginning subluxation-coxarthrosis; Chiari pelvic osteotomy. Ten years later very good remodeling of the acetabular roof with good sphericity and satisfactory joint space

sidered, as these young adults do not seek medical attention because of pain, but for radiologic and clinical evidence of coxarthrosis. These factors are indications for surgical intervention. Clinical results are therefore somewhat misleading. Ten years after surgery, one observes a persistent marked improvement of the patients' gait pattern and an astonishing non-progression of the coxarthrosis. The reason for this is the remodeling of the acetabular roof (Fig. 1).

Radiological Results

Evaluation of radiologic results is also not easy. Coxometry is of little value. For example, the CE angle (Wiberg) may be identical in different situations depending on the height and slope of the osteotomy, but results can be totally different (Fig. 2). Therefore one has

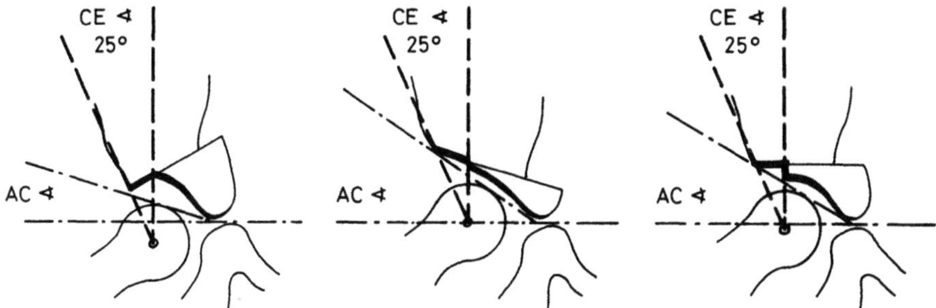

Fig. 2. The CE angle can be similar in spite of different shapes of the acetabular roof, depending on height and direction of the pelvic osteotomy

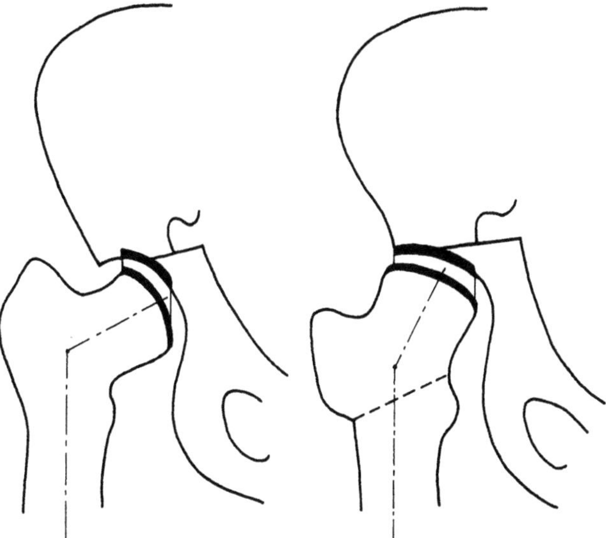

Fig. 3. In cases of subluxation-coxarthrosis combined with a deformed femoral head, pelvic osteotomy alone is insufficient. Simultaneous valgus osteotomy enlarges the weight bearing joint surface

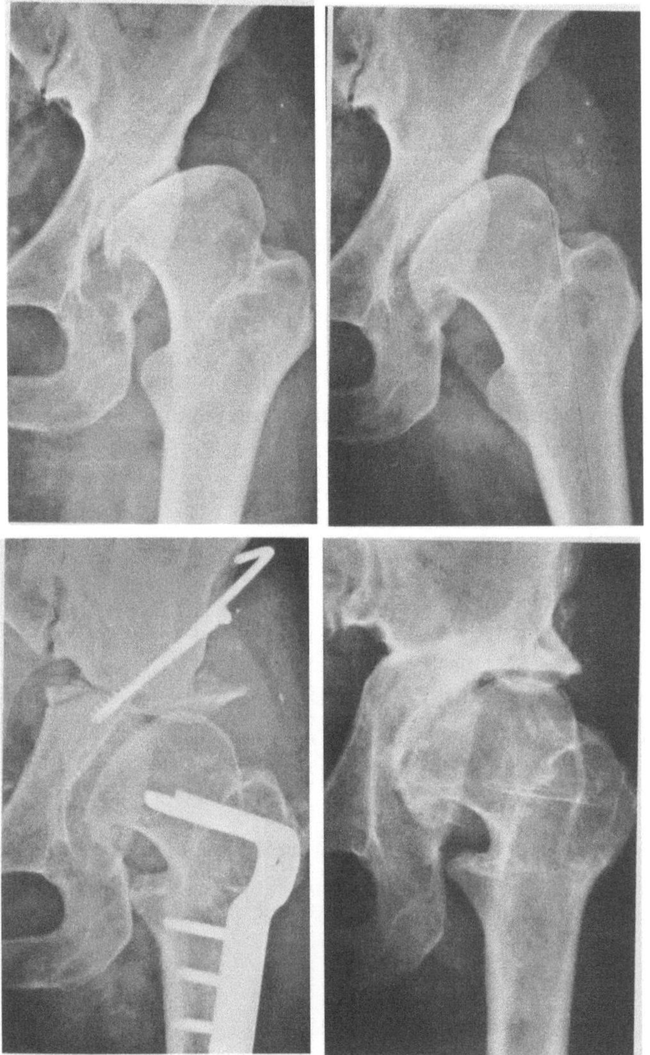

Fig. 4. J.P. b. 1926. 34 years old patient with subluxation-coxarthrosis and ovoid femoral head. Marked improvement after Chiari – and slight valgus osteotomy. Ventral gap has been filled with a bone graft removed from the valgus osteotomy site. Course during an 11 year period

to evaluate joint congruency and findings of arthrosis, particularly joint space diminution and sclerosis of the acetabular roof. In considering these factors, one will note that in 4/5 of the cases arthrotic findings are less evident or unchanged 10 years after surgery. Only in less than 1/5 of hips did we observe an increase of arthrotic findings 10 years postoperatively.

One has to consider the necessity for an intertrochanteric osteotomy if the indication for pelvic osteotomy includes cases of more or less developed subluxation-coxarthrosis. As already stated, preoperative functional X-rays are required to predetermine optimum enlargement of the weight bearing joint surface. One should not be influenced by a certain amount of cranial displacement observed in cases of a subluxating coxa valga with adduction. Better joint surface congruity at the craniolateral sector is provided by a valgus osteotomy. The contact area will be supported by a pelvic osteotomy. Varus osteotomy would result in a smaller contact area caudal to the pelvic osteotomy site (Figs. 3 and 4).

Discussion and Conclusion

Results of Chiari pelvic osteotomy performed on older adolescents and young adults in the presence of pre-existing coxarthrosis continue to be encouraging 10 years after surgery. Clinical results are better than the impression gained by employing Merle d'Aubi-

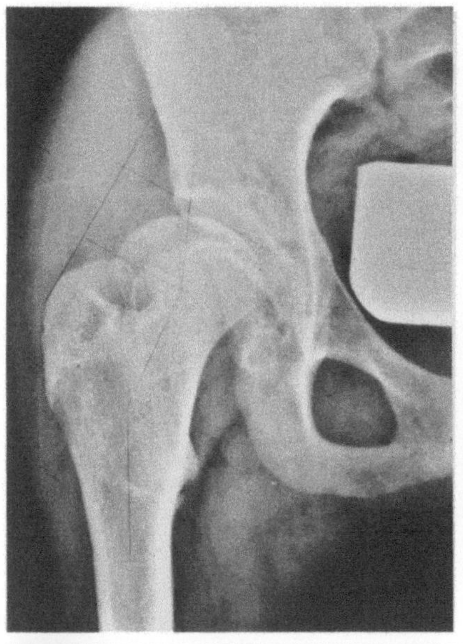
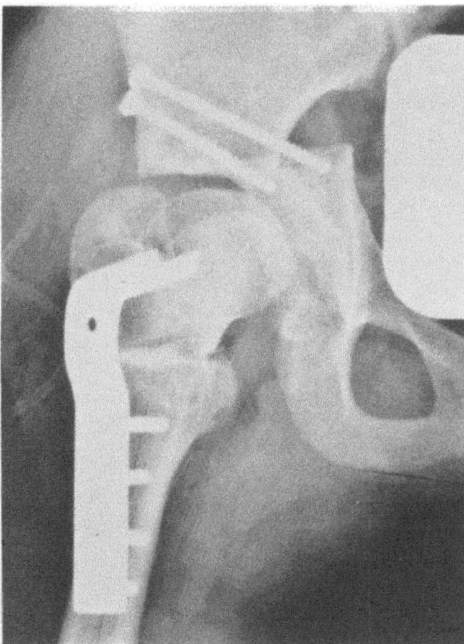
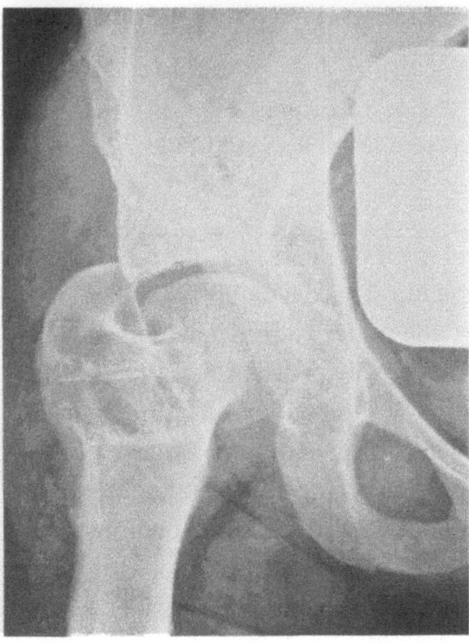

Fig. 5. A.L. b. 1952. 14 year old patient. Level pelvic osteotomy. Spherical adaptation of the acetabular roof and the femoral head 8 years after surgery

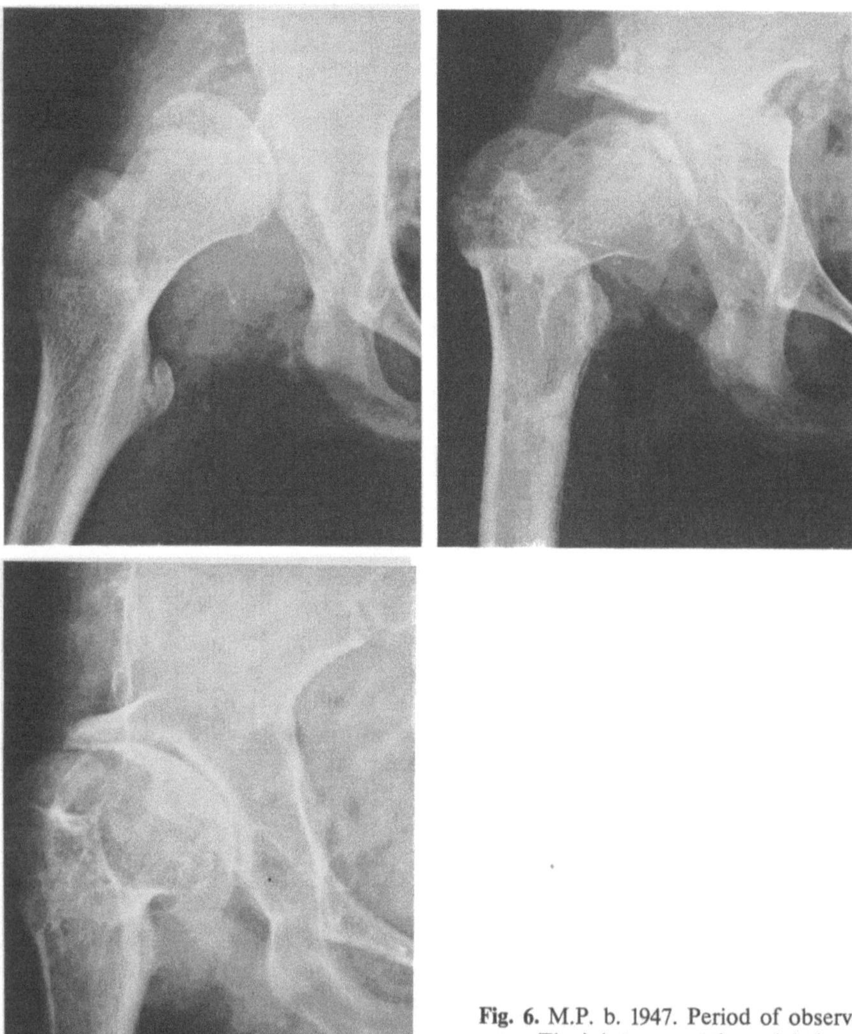

Fig. 6. M.P. b. 1947. Period of observation 19 years. The joint space at the weight bearing sector remains well-preserved in spite of femoral head deformation. Patient is free of pain

gné's point system of hip joint evaluation, particularly if one considers the rapid deterioration of untreated subluxation-coxarthrosis of the hip. This development can be arrested in more than half of the cases. Radiologically one notices improvement or non-progression in 4/5 of the patients 10 years postoperatively. Less than 1/5 of the hips show signs of deterioration. The arrest of the deterioration of subluxation-coxarthrosis in contrast to untreated cases is particularly impressive when the patients' improved gait pattern is observed. Therefore we have increased our indications for this operation during the last few years. In cases of advanced subluxation-coxarthrosis one has to combine pelvic with intertrochanteric osteotomy. A valgus osteotomy will usually be required as it alone guaranties enlargement of the weight bearing joint surfaces. Since 1972 we have completely abandoned the Chiari pelvic osteotomy for children with dysplastic hips prior to the age of 6, except for cases with a very steep and small acetabular roof. We recommend keeping the operation as simple as possible. For this reason we employ a level osteotomy in an ascending direction from dorsolateral to ventromedial. In this manner, it is possible to carry out a satisfactory displacement of the bony parts and to provide good ventral support with a bone graft obtained from the iliac crest or the intertrochanteric area in cases of simultaneous intertrochanteric osteotomy. Adaptive functional processes even after cessation of bone growth and in the presence of preexisting coxarthrosis remodel the acetabular roof and result in unexpectedly satisfactory joint congruency during the postoperative period (Figs. 5 and 6).

Summary

Experiences gained in over 500 Chiari pelvic osteotomies and reexaminations 10 or more years after surgery performed on preschool children and on patients after cessation of bone growth have changed our indications for this operation. As of this date we hardly ever perform it on children with hip dysplasia under the age of 6. An increasing number of older adolescents and young adults are now treated with this method, even in the presence of a subluxation-coxarthrosis. More than one half of these patients had a simultaneous or second stage intertrochanteric osteotomy. A higher degree of coxarthrosis requires intertrochanteric osteotomy more frequently. In most cases this will have to be a valgus osteotomy to obtain optimum enlargement of the weight bearing joint surfaces. Functional adaptive mechanisms acting on the acetabular roof result in astonishingly good congruency of the hip joint components during the postoperative period.

References

Ieda H, Winkler W (1979) Langzeitergebnisse der Beckenosteotomie nach Chiari durchgeführt an Kindern im Vorschulalter. Orthopäde 8: 44–48
Schreiber A (1976) Ostéotomie du bassin selon Chiari. Rev Chir Orthop 62:569
Winkler W, Weber A (1977) Beckenosteotomie nach Chiari. Z Orthop 115:167

Translation from the German: Schreiber A (1979) Langzeitergebnisse der Beckenosteotomie nach Chiari beim Erwachsenen. Orthopäde 8:264–268. © Springer Verlag 1979

Results of Intertrochanteric Osteotomies in Patients with Coxarthrosis 12–15 Years After Surgery

R. Schneider

From September 1959 to June 1962, we performed 109 intertrochanteric osteotomies on 100 patients. Their average age was 59 years. Every patient was re-examined 2–5, 7, and 12–15 years postoperatively.

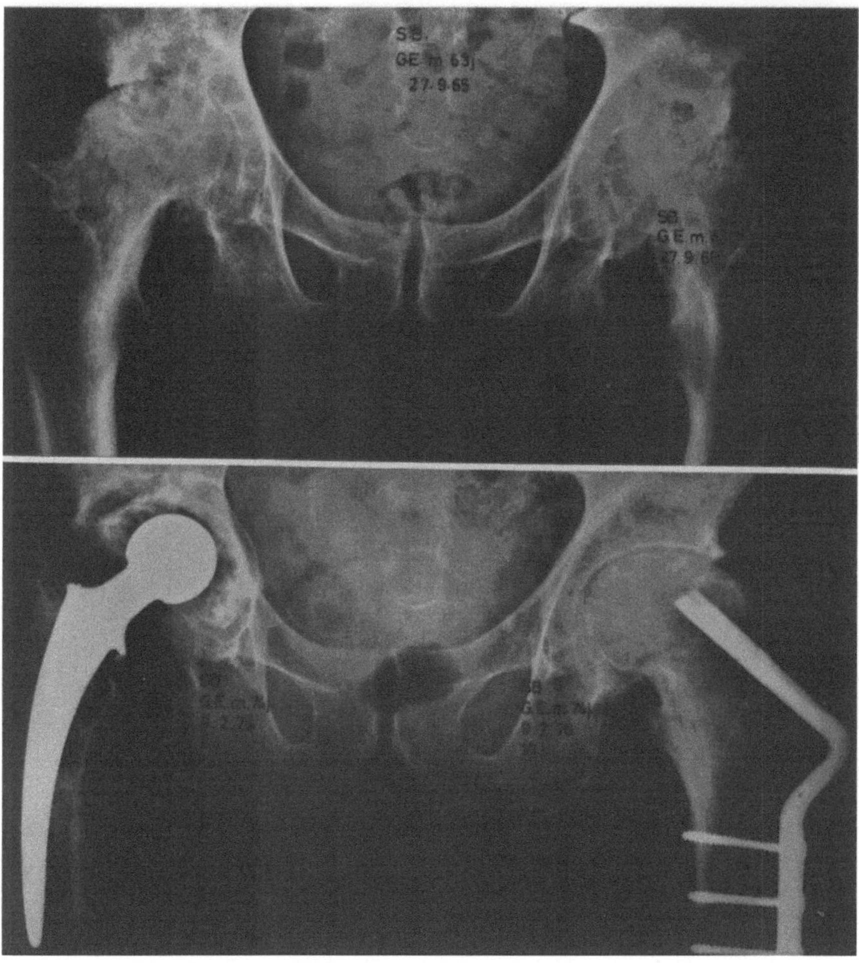

Fig. 1. Above: Farmer, 63 years old. Marked bilateral coxarthrosis 1965. Below: 10 years after intertrochanteric osteotomy, left hip. Perfect joint regeneration. Patient is clinically symptom free. Right: Total hip prothesis is unstable

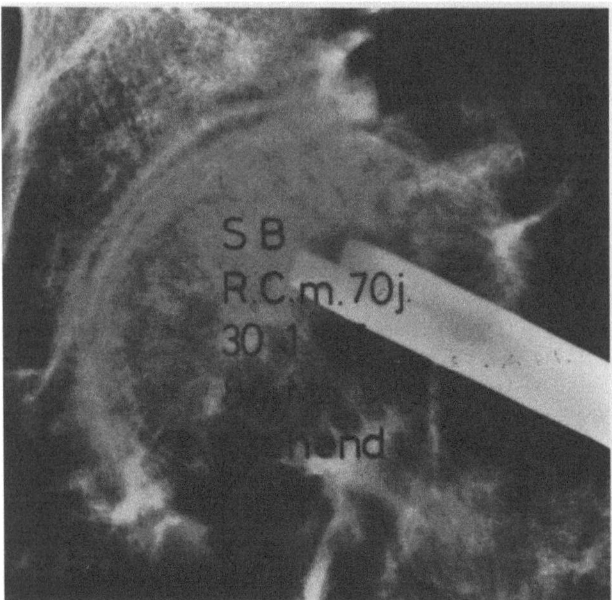

Fig. 2. Arthographic demonstration of newly formed cartilage of the acetabulum and the femoral head. Same patient as demonstrated in Fig. 3

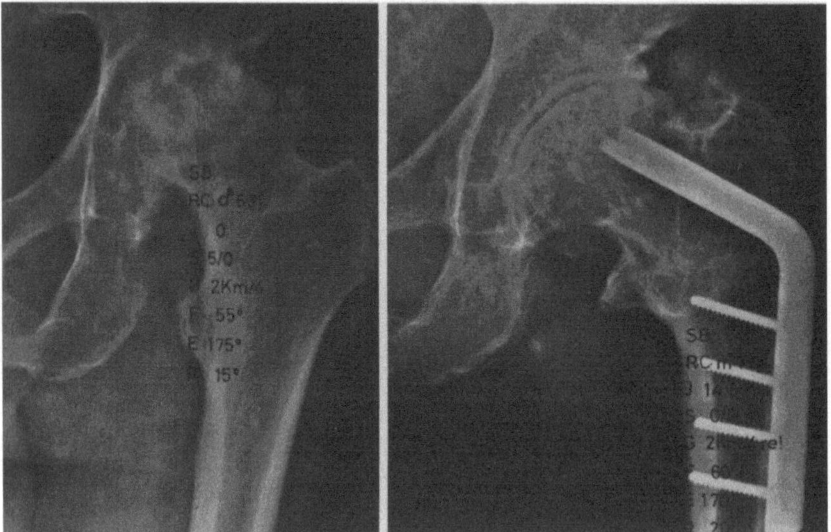

Fig. 3. Farmer 63 years old. Improved joint condition persists 15 years after surgery

I would like to present the case of a 63 year old farmer (Fig. 1) to demonstrate the beneficial effects of intertrochanteric osteotomy in the age of total joint replacement. Severe bilateral coxarthrosis with loss of the joint space was present in 1965. A left intertrochanteric osteotomy was performed in 1965, a right total hip joint replacement was carried out in 1970. In 1976, ten years after the intertrochanteric osteotomy, the left hip joint was found to be fully functional and pain free. X-rays showed regeneration with a congruent 3 mm wide joint space. Six years after implantation of the artificial hip joint one notices

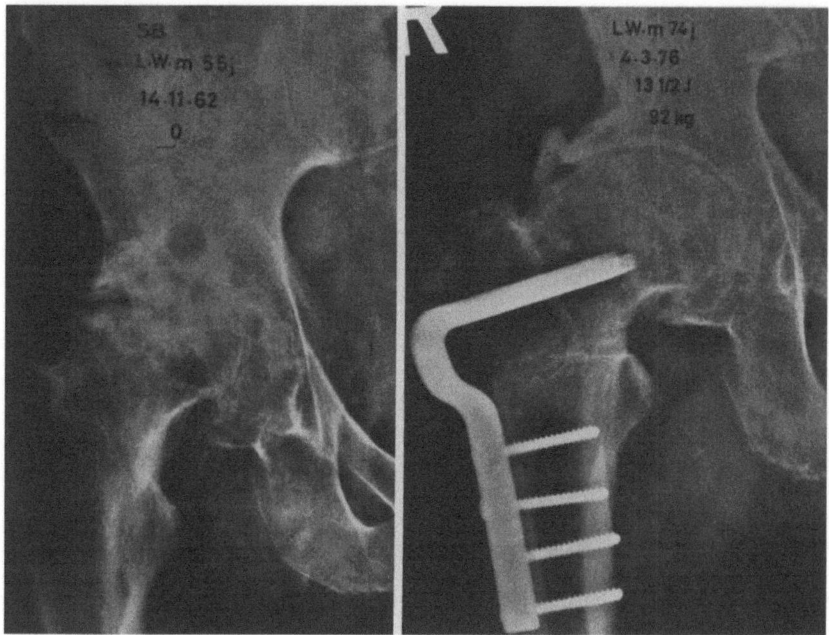

Fig. 4. Contractor, 55 years old. Left: Marked joint destruction. Right: Joint regeneration maintained, 90° flexion 14 years after surgery

loosening of the prothesis, resulting in pain. The progress of the patient's left hip is truly remarkable if one considers the condition of the right hip before and after the total hip joint replacement.

The basis for joint remodeling is the newly formed cartilage on both joint surfaces. An arthrogram (Fig. 2) proves this fact. Five years later, the left hip joint showed no signs of further deterioration (Fig. 3).

In the presence of relatively healthy bone, slight improvement of biomechanical conditions of the hip seems to be sufficient to interrupt the vicious cycle of destruction and to start a period of reconstruction. The case of a contractor weighing 90 Kg gives additional proof of this statement (Fig. 4). Fourteen years after surgery, the hip continues to be fully functional and without pain.

Intertrochanteric osteotomy is indicated even in the presence of complete loss of motion with marked malposition of the hip joint. Two cases of adduction-flexion deformity were corrected by varus-extension osteotomy. Both patients were unable to flex their hips prior to surgery. Thirteen years later, both patients are pain free and were able to flex their hips by 60° and 70° respectively. X-rays showed definite improvement of the joint space (Fig. 5).

Reexamination of every patient in our series 12–15 years postoperatively revealed the following results: One third was rated as good (average age 69 years), one third was deceased and one third was regarded to have poor results, as they required reoperations after a median period of eight years.

Questionnaires sent to relatives of our deceased patients showed that the condition of 27 of 31 patients' hips remained good or satisfactory.

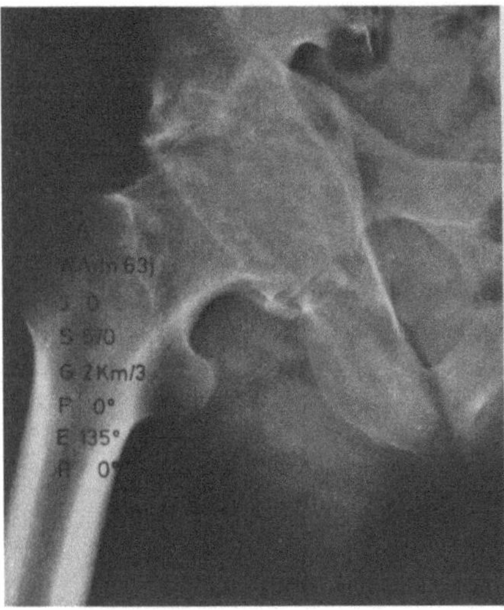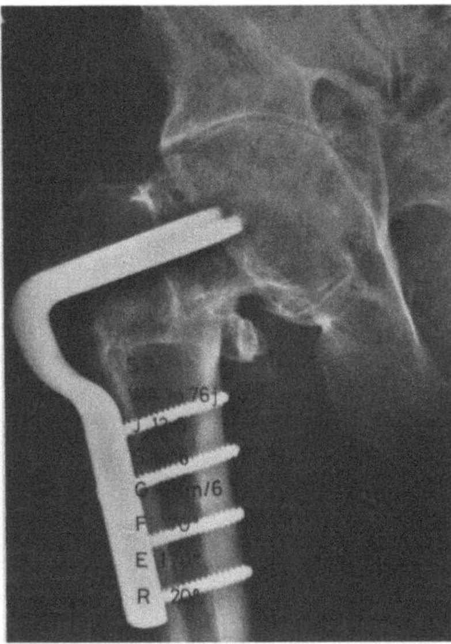

Fig. 5. Farmer, 63 years old. Left: Hip is fixed in adduction and flexion. Painful primary coxarthrosis. Right: 13 years after corrective osteotomy. Painless hip joint, flexion increased by 70°, rotation by 20°. Flexion contracture reduced from 45° to 10°

A breakdown of the 38 hips requiring reoperation after a median period of eight years reduces this number if one considers that many patients in this group had a satisfactory result five years after initial surgery.

The two tables summarize our results (Tables 1 and 2). The results were obtained with varus-, valgus- and simple displacement osteotomies. 60% of our patients required an additional extension osteotomy of approximately 30%.

It is impossible to draw conclusions with regard to the particular value of each osteotomy type, as their results depend on proper indication. Indications for intertrochanteric osteotomy were set extremely widely during the period of our investigative series. Functional analysis of long term results shows that rotation increases after surgery. This increase continues to improve further between the 7th–14th postoperative year. Improv-

Table 1. Results of 100 patients with coxarthrosis treated by 109 intertrochanteric osteotomies 12–15 years after surgery

		Pat	Op
I Reexaminations	good or satisfactory	33	37
	poor	2	
II Deceased (without reoperation – from questionnaire)	good or satisfactory	27	34
	poor	4	
III Poor results (with reoperation approx. 8 years postoperatively		34	38
34 total hip joint replacements 4 arthrodeses			

Table 2. Types of surgery: 108 operations

	Valg.	Var.	Displ.	Add. Ext.	Total
I Reexamined 25 females, 10 males	13	20	4	23	37
II Deceased 27 females, 4 males	13	10	11	23	34
III Reoperation 34 total hip joint replacement 4 arthrodeses	20	17	1	20	38

Explanation: Valg.   = Valgus osteotomy
Var.   = Varus osteotomy
Displ.   = Displacement osteotomy
Add. Ext. = Additional extension osteotomy

ed rotation corresponds with decrease of pain. Rotational position, extension and lower limb length is not affected by time. Lack of pain prevents relapse into malposition. Range of flexion is not improved by surgery, but it did not decrease during the observation period. Increase of flexion was noted in individual cases, but loss of flexion was noted occasionally even in good results.

Conclusion

In spite of generous indications for intertrochanteric osteotomy, we observed good satisfactory results in nearly one half of our patients 12–15 years after initial surgery.

Translation from the German: Schneider R (1979) 12–15 Jahres-Resultate nach intertrochanterer Osteotomie bei Coxarthrose. Orthopäde 8:79–82 © Springer Verlag 1979

Long Term Results of Acetabular Shelf Arthroplasty

J. Judet and H. Judet

This paper is based on recent examinations of 655 hips treated by acetabular shelf arthroplasty at least 10 years ago (median observation period − 16 years).

All patients were reexamined on the occasion of a report presented to the French Orthopaedic Association (SOFCOT) in 1975. They were treated in different orthopaedic departments in Paris and throughout France.

Material and Method

Long term evaluation of acetabular shelf arthroplasty requires definition of the anatomic anomalies and the grade of severity of arthrotic changes employed as pertinent criteria.

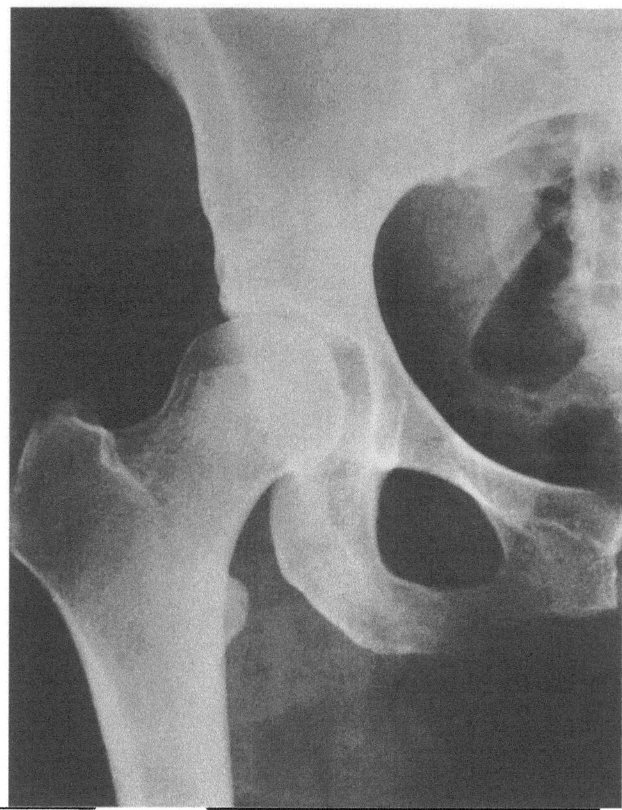

Fig. 1. Pure acetabular dysplasia

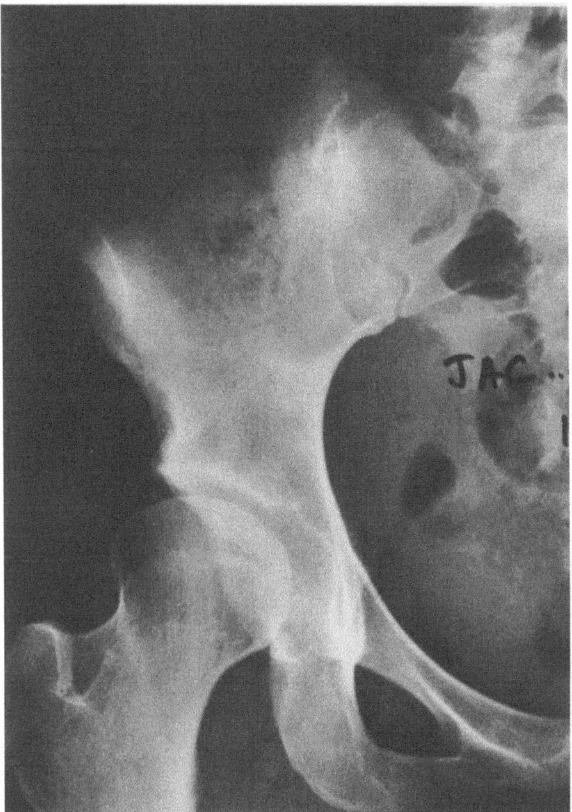

Fig. 2. Acetabular dysplasia with coxa valga

We distinguished 4 basic anatomic anomalies:
1. *Pure acetabular dysplasia* (Fig. 1): Normal CCD angle, but with a very small CE angle (Wiberg) of less than 20° (22% of our cases belonged to this group).
2. *Acetabular dysplasia with coxa valga* (Fig. 2): The CCD angle is larger than 135°; the acetabular deformity is similar to 1. (13% of all cases).
3. *Congenital subluxation* (Fig. 3): The acetabulum is not only dysplastic but also displaced; Menard-Shentons line is always interrupted; the head is more or less decentralized (52% of all cases).
4. *Congenital dislocation* (Fig. 4): The acetabulum is totally deformed; markedly increased valgus position of head and neck is noted (13% of all cases).

We consequently distinguished 3 grades of severity of arthrotic changes at the time of initial surgery:
1. *No arthrotic changes* (30%) of cases: Normal joint space; no osteophytes; no bony sclerosis.
2. *Early arthrotic changes* (Fig. 5) (42%) of cases: Joint space diminished, but its width is still one half larger than normal. Moderate osteophyte formation; evidence of discreet bony sclerosis.

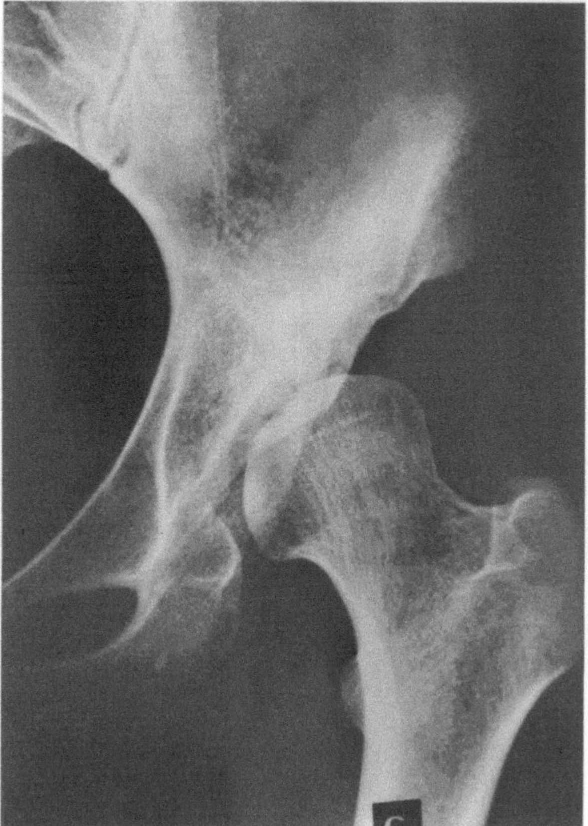

Fig. 3. Congenital subluxation

3. *Advanced arthrotic changes* (Fig. 6) (28%) of cases: Joint space diminished to less than one half of the norm. Evidence of a triangular lateral acetabular area with excessive weight bearing and bony sclerosis; osteophyte formation.

The percentage figures show that the 2 largest groups consist of cases with subluxation and with early arthrotic changes. They represent the classical indication for acetabular shelf arthroplasty.

Results

As a first step the results were evaluated in toto. Then they were broken down according to the above mentioned criteria.

The total figures revealed that, after a median observation period of 16 years, postoperative results were good in 64%, acceptable in 19% and poor in 17% of cases. According to radiological evidence, 2% improved, 65% showed no change and 33% deteriorated.

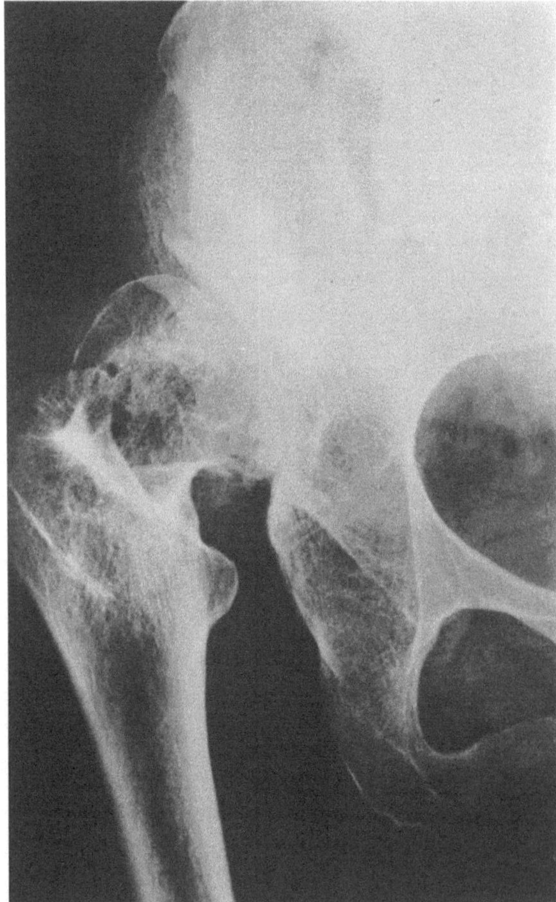

Fig. 4. Congenital hip dislocation

If the results were classified by age, amount of arthrosis and length of observation, we noted that
– operations performed after the fourth decade of life were less successful
– operations performed in the presence of arthrotic changes were less successful
– rapid deterioration of postoperative success occurred 17–20 years after surgery (Table 1).

Results in different anatomic anomaly groups:
Good results were observed in 72% of hips with pure dysplasia, poor results in 7% (Fig. 7). Success lasted for a longer period, deterioration began 20 years postoperatively. Results in patients with dysplasia combined with coxa valga were essentially similar. It was also our impression that their tendency to deteriorate was less pronounced even in cases of advanced arthrosis.

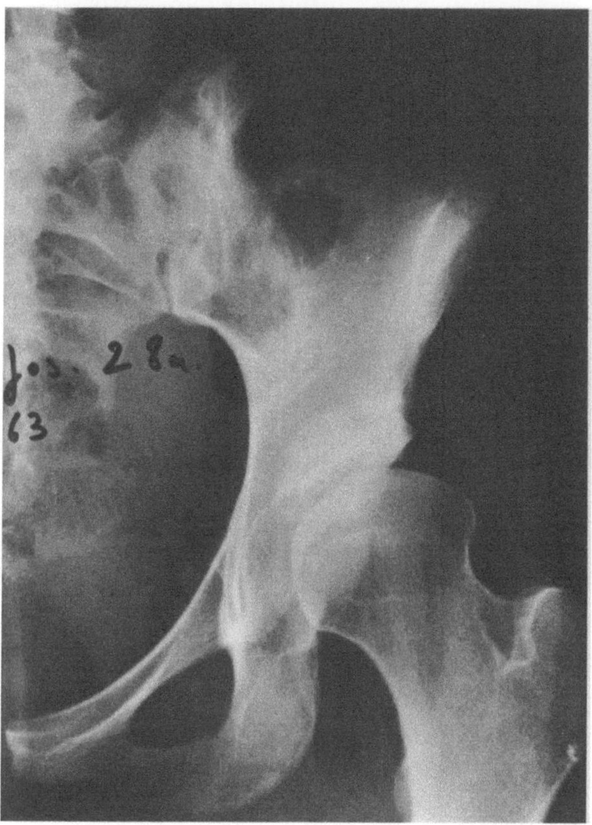

Fig. 5. Early arthrotic changes

Results in patients with hip subluxation were judged to be good in 60% and poor in 24% of cases. Rapid deterioration began 15 years after surgery (Fig. 8), but advanced arthrotic changes were frequently present at the time of initial surgery.

Results in patients with hip dislocation were good in 59% of cases. Surgery performed after the fourth decade of life resulted in a rapid decline of cases with satisfactory outcome (Fig. 9).

Our analysis clearly shows that certain anatomic anomalies respond better to surgical intervention than others, but that the success rate was never below 59%. We therefore believe that acetabular shelf arthroplasty has a wide indication.

We were also interested to determine if acetabular shelf arthroplasty is an operation of preventive nature in regard to development of arthrosis. To answer this question, we re-examined 168 dysplastic hip joints, which showed no signs of arthrosis at the time of surgery.

The 86% quota of good results noted in this group was definitely higher when compared with the total average. The same percentage showed no radiological signs of deterioration. Even now, 15 or more years after surgery, no evidence of arthrosis is present. Many of these patients (one third) are now older than 45 years. In this age group signs of secondary arthrosis are commonly noted in patients with hip dysplasia. Therefore it was our impression that acetabular shelf arthroplasty retards the development of arthrosis.

Surgery is indicated *only* in cases with functional impairment, particularly in the presence of pain. We have *never* performed an acetabular shelf arthroplasty on dysplastic hips *in the absence* of clinical symptoms or radiologic findings or arthrosis.

Discussion

Acetabular shelf arthroplasty is a satisfactory procedure with a high rate of success. Depending on anatomic anomalies, one can expect good results in 60%–75% of cases after a median observation period of 16 years.

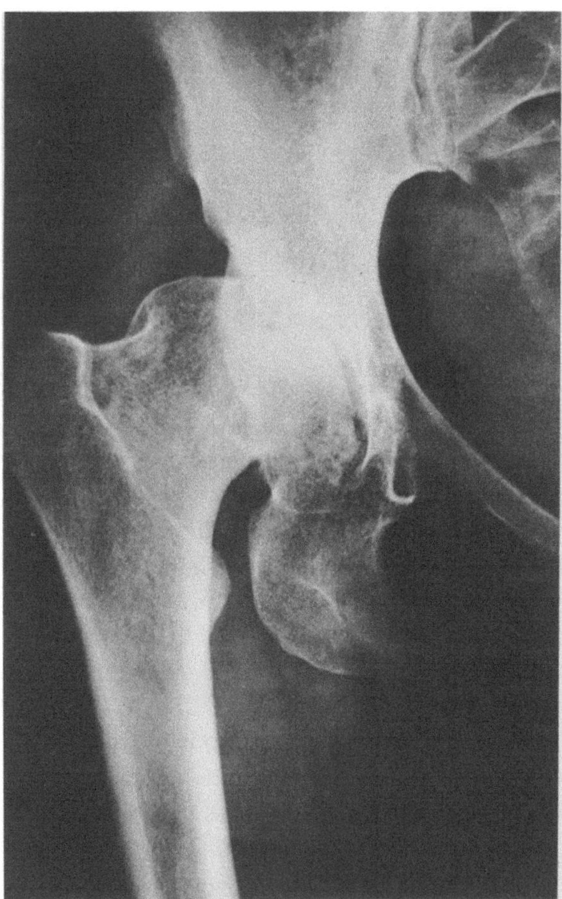

Fig. 6. Advanced arthrotic changes

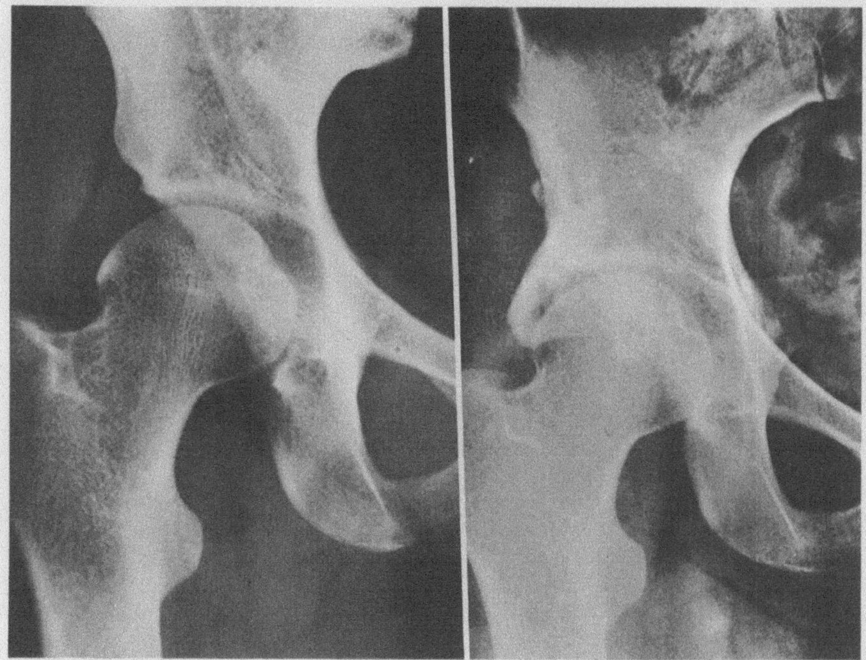

Fig. 7. Good result in a case of pure acetabular dysplasia. Right: Well preserved joint space, no arthrotic changes 20 years post-operatively. Left: Preoperative condition

In the compass of surgery to correct congenital malalignment of the hip, acetabular shelf arthroplasty takes its place with varus or valgus osteotomy and the Chiari pelvic osteotomy.

The *advantages* of acetabular shelf arthroplasty are:
– the relative technical ease of the operation
– the low incidence of postoperative complications.

Table 1. Influence of time on deterioration of results

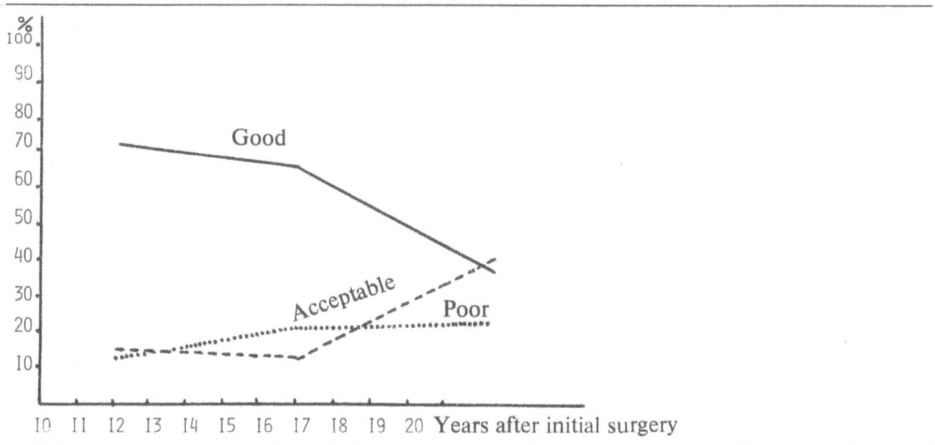

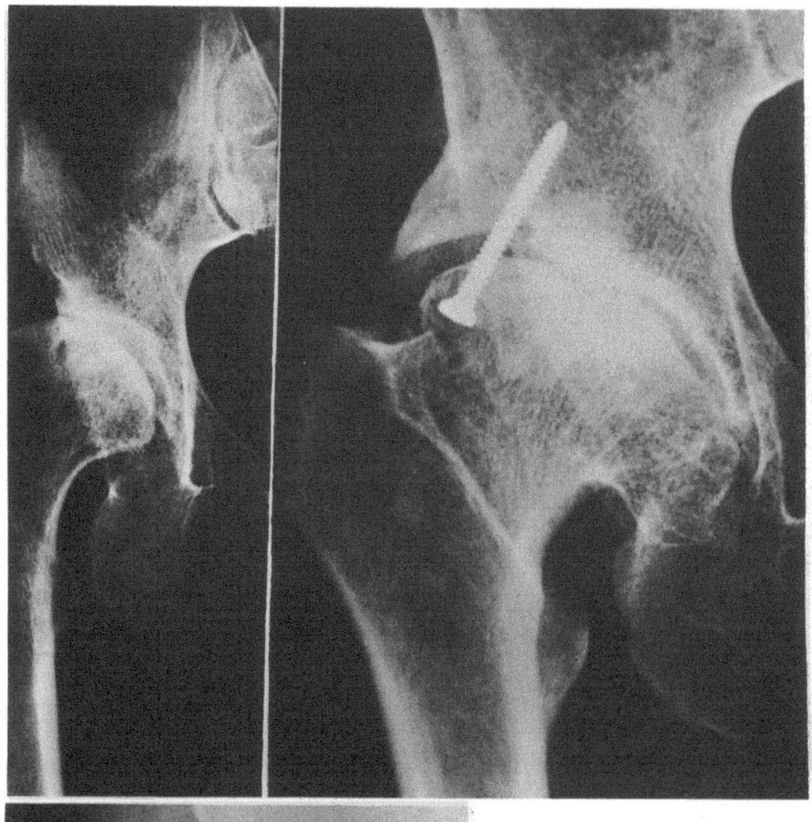
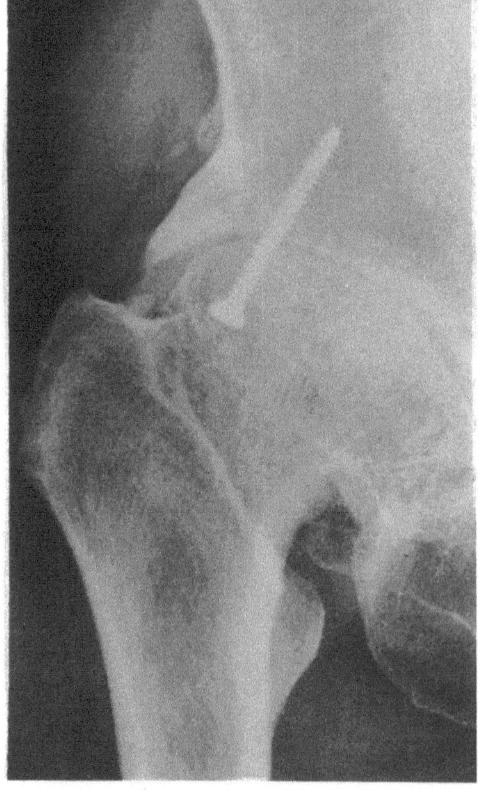

Fig. 8. Good result in a case of subluxation and advanced arthrotic changes. Top left: Preoperative condition, marked arthrotic changes. Top right: 1 year after acetabular shelf arthroplasty. Markedly diminished joint space, persistent evidence of abnormal wear. Bottom left: 18 years later: Improved joint space and less abnormal wear

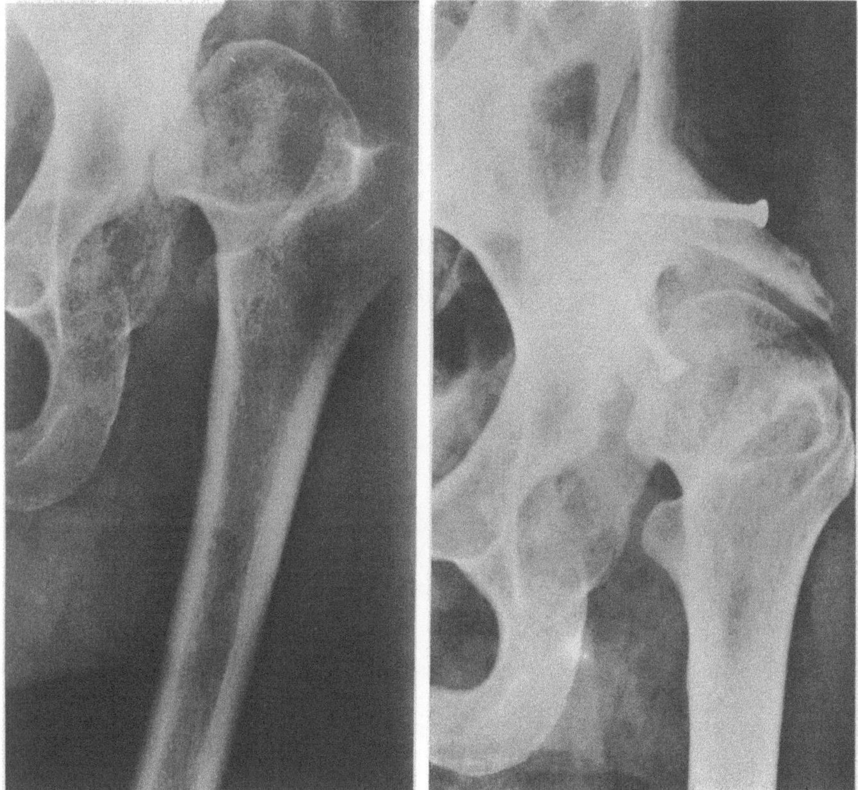

Fig. 9. Good result in a case of dislocation 18 years after surgery. Left: Preoperative condition. Right: 18 years later

This type of surgery does not shorten the involved lower limb and the pelvic diameter is not diminished, in contrast to varus or Chiari pelvic osteotomies.

The surface of the acetabulum is enlarged, an important factor if a second operation has to be considered, i.e. a total hip joint replacement.

The *value* of the operation is *limited* by the facts that normal functional conditions cannot be recreated, joint congruency obtainable with an intertrochanteric osteotomy cannot be achieved, or medialisation, as in pelvic osteotomy (Chiari) cannot be obtained.

Results in patients without arthrotic chances are remarkable (82% good). The operation also seems to have a preventative function in retarding development of arthrotic changes.

The operation can still be considered for patients with early arthrotic changes (72% good), but in the presence of severe arthrosis MacMurray osteotomy or total hip joint replacement for patients of the proper age group may be indicated.

For patients with acetabular dysplasia combined with coxa valga and for subluxation we recommend varus osteotomies; in cases where dysplasia dominates, one may consider combining shelf arthroplasty and intertrochanteric osteotomy (Fig. 10). Acetabular

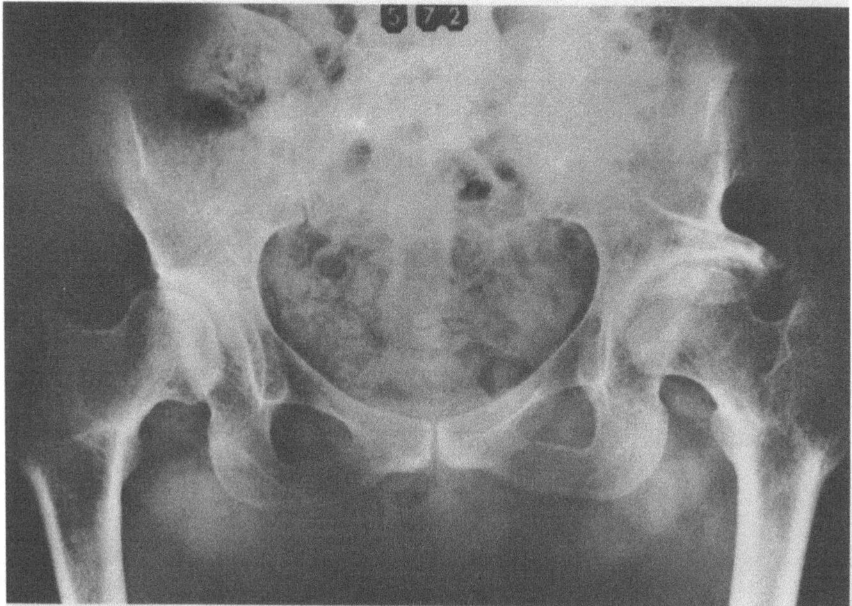

Fig. 10. Acetabular dysplasia with coxa valga. Right: Varus osteotomy combined with acetabular shelf arthroplasty. Head coverage is better, its varus position is more physiologic. Left: Varus osteotomy only. The femoral head is located in the acetabulum but only incompletely covered, particularly its anterior segment. Marked varus position was required at the time of initial surgery

shelf arthroplasty loses much of its effectiveness in the presence of advanced arthrosis, therefore it is only indicated if arthrotic changes are minimal.

Patients with dislocation or with subluxation with marked or total loss of bony femoral head coverage are better treated with a pelvic osteotomy. An acetabular shelf athroplasty will not provide satisfactory coverage for the femoral head by the deformed acetabulum.

Conclusion

Acetabular shelf arthroplasty promises good results for patients with hip dysplasia combined with slight arthrotic changes. It can be successful in young patients with subluxation combined with slight arthrotic changes.

Frequently it can be combined with a varus osteotomy in the presence of pronounced dysplasia.

It is our opinion that acetabular shelf arthroplasty continues to be of great value as a joint preserving operation for patients with dysplastic hip joints.

Summary

655 hips treated by acetabular shelf arthroplasty were examined and evaluated. Their mean observation period after surgery was 16 years (minimum 10 years). The results were analysed according to 4 basic anatomic anomalies and 3 grades of arthrotic severity.

2/3 of the hips were judged to be good 10 years postoperatively. In general, deterioration started 17–20 years after initial surgery.

Surgery performed after the fourth decade of life and early arthrotic changes are factors which impair our results.

References

Judet J (1976) Résultats des butées cotyloidinnes ayant 10 ans on plus de recul. Symposium de la SOFCOT. Rev Chir Orthop 62:511–577

Translation from the German: Judet H (1979) Ergebnisse der Pfannendachplastik nach mehr als 10 Jahren. Orthopäde 8:269–275 © Springer Verlag 1979

Treatment of Osteoarthritis of the Knee by Osteotomy

P. Maquet

The antero-posterior X-ray of a normal knee demonstrates an even thickness of sub-chondral sclerosis under each tibial plateau (Fig. 2a). As Pauwels [10] has shown, the quantity of bone tissue is proportional to the mechanical stresses. Greater stresses provoke deposition of bone, smaller stresses resorption. Therefore, the shape of the sub-chondral sclerosis corresponds to that of the stress diagram or load distribution curve. From the pattern of even thickness of the subchondral sclerosis under the tibial plateau, we can conclude that the stresses are evenly distributed in a normal knee. Since the weight bearing area of the medial and lateral plateau are approximately equal [9], the overall force acting on the joint is thus exerted at the centre of gravity of the weight bearing surfaces which occurs at the centre of the knee (Fig 1).

During the unilateral stance in gait, the knee eccentrically bears the body minus the supporting lower leg and foot [8]. The force P due to this partial body mass tends to tilt the femur in adduction on the tibia. Force P acts with a lever arm a which is the distance between the line of action of P and the centre G of the knee.

Force P is counterbalanced by a muscular force L which acts with the lever arm b, the distance between G and the line of action of L. The force L developed by the muscles directly opposed to force P, in relation to G, is successively anterolateral, lateral and postero-lateral during the unilateral stance in gait [9].

The resultant R is the vectorial sum of the forces P and L. It is transmitted from femur to tibia through weight bearing surfaces which vary with the movement of the joint as does force R. These weight bearing surfaces include the menisci. The weight bearing surfaces are largest in full extension and diminish by about 50% when the menisci are removed.

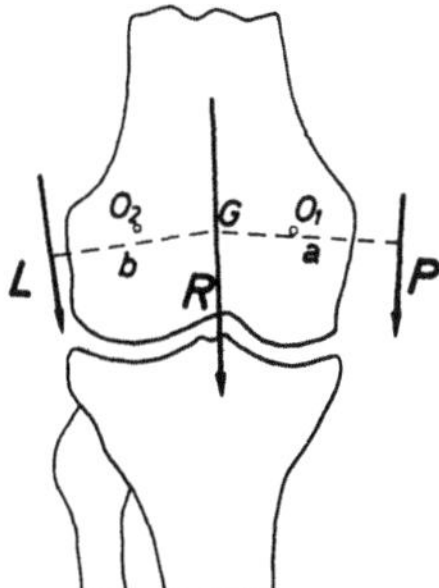

Fig. 1

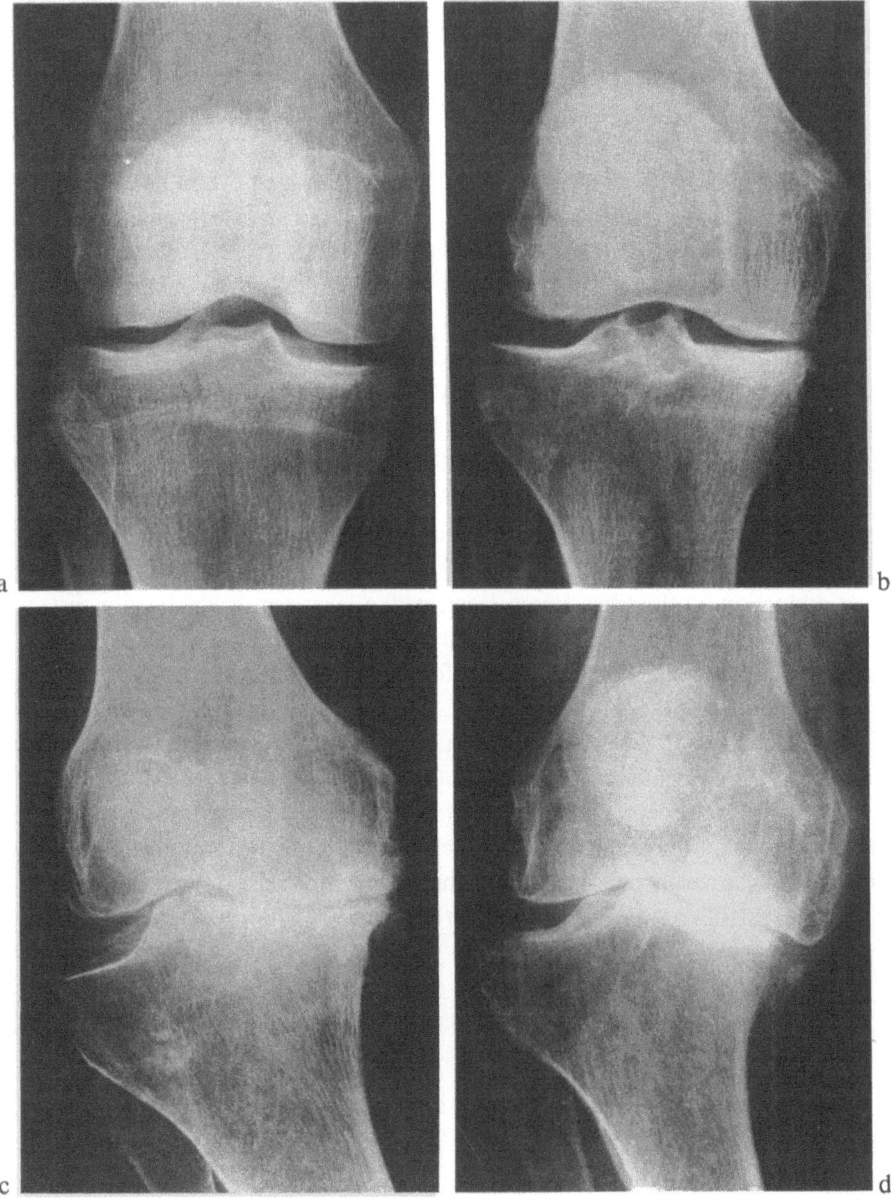

Fig. 2a–d

Force R provokes compressive stresses in the joint. Their magnitude and distribution depend on the overall force R and on the weight bearing surfaces of the joint. As mentioned above, they are evenly distributed over the weight bearing surfaces of a normal knee (Fig 2a). The greater the force R, the greater the articular compressive stresses become. If the weight bearing surfaces of the joint are reduced, the articular compressive stresses increase correspondingly.

In osteoarthritis of the medial aspect of the knee, the subchondral sclerosis increases under the medial tibial plateau and tends to fade away under the lateral. A dense triangle appears under the medial plateau (Fig 2b). The medial joint space becomes narrowed and then disappears while the subchondral sclerosis further increases (Fig 2c). Finally the resistance of the bony tissue is overwhelmed. Bone is resorbed and the femur subluxates on the tibia (Fig. 2d).

The alteration of the subchondral sclerosis corresponds to a modification of the stress diagram in the joint and to a medial displacement of the resultant R. Such a medial displacement of force R can be caused:
− by a weakening of the muscles L;
− by an increase of the body weight if this is not compensated by a corresponding increase of force L;
− by a varus deformity of the leg;
− by a horizontal displacement of the centre of gravity of the body away from the knee [9].

Of these different possibilities, weakening of the lateral muscles was found in all the cases of osteoarthritis of the knee with a varus deformity which Blaimont subjected to measurement [1].

Medial displacement of force R causes an asymmetrical distribution of the compressive stresses which are then increased and concentrated in the medial compartment of the joint. There the articular cartilage is destroyed. Destruction of the cartilage causes or increases a varus deformity. This displaces the resultant R further medially, which in turn increases the compressive stresses in the medial compartment of the knee. A vicious circle is thus created.

In osteoarthritis of the lateral aspect of the knee, one observes a more marked cancellous structure and an increased sclerosis under the lateral plateau (Fig 3a). The area of sclerosis is cup-shaped and localized in the centre of the plateau. At a later stage it increases in size and moves towards the intercondylar eminence while the lateral joint space becomes narrower (Fig 3b). Finally the femur subluxates on the tibia. The valgus deformity thus increases, the medial joint space opens up and the cancellous structure tends to fade away under the medial plateau (Fig. 3c). These signs demonstrate a lateral displacement of resultant R. It can be displaced laterally either by an increase of force L a valgus deformity, or a horizontal displacement of the centre of gravity S_7 towards the knee [8, 9].

An increase of the muscular force L, undesirable for the knee, may be necessary to ensure equilibrium at hip level since some of the muscles developing force L are biarticular, bridging both the hip and the knee.

Lateral displacement of resultant R concentrates the compressive stresses in the lateral compartment of the knee rather in the vicinity of the intercondylar eminence because of the direction of R (Fig. 3). The local concentration and uneven distribution of the stresses provoke destruction of the articular cartilage. Therefore, the lateral joint space is narrowed and a valgus deformity appears or increases. This in turn displaces the resultant R further laterally, additionally increasing the compressive stresses in the joint. Again this is a vicious circle.

The distribution of the articular stresses can also be read on the lateral X-rays. Whereas the plateaux of a normal knee are underlined by a subchondral sclerosis of even thick-

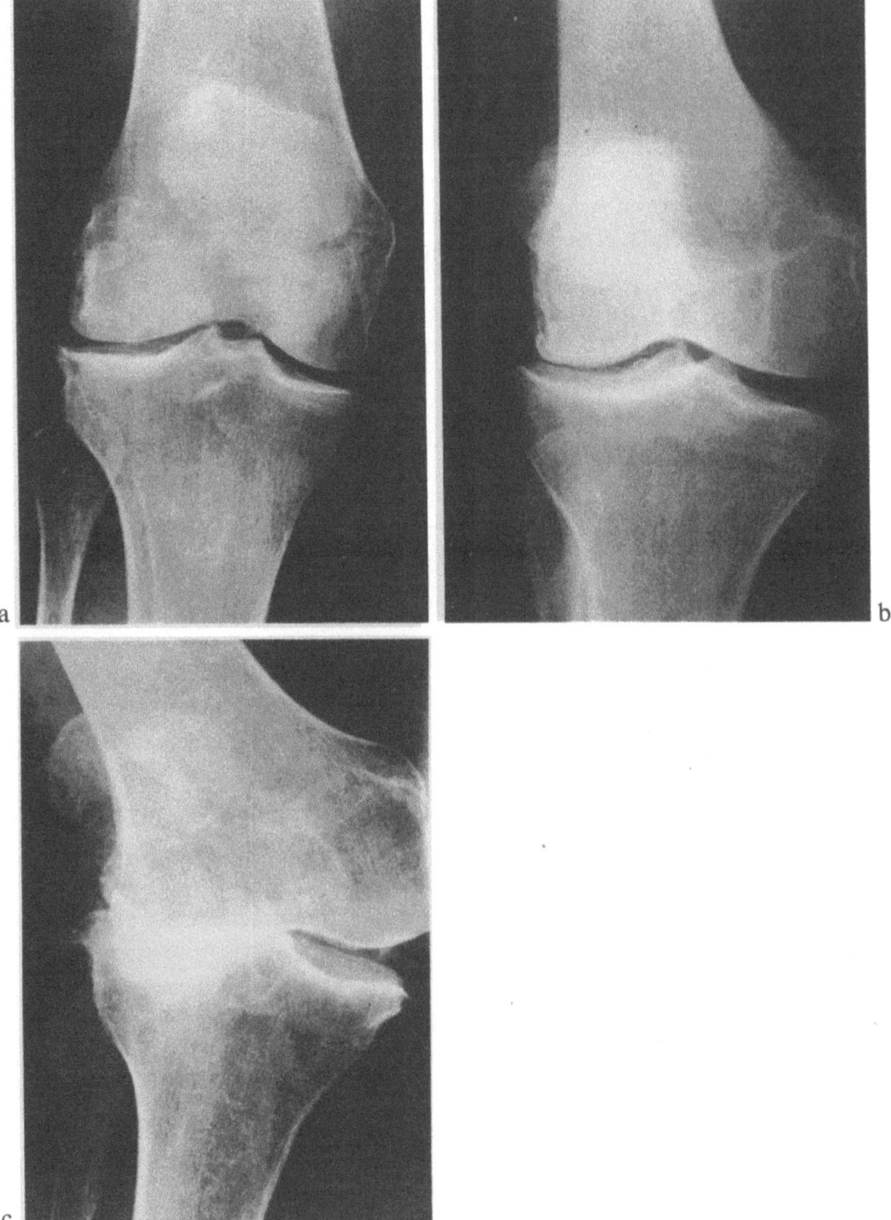

Fig. 3a–c

ness throughout (Fig. 4a), in a knee with a flexion contracture a sclerotic triangle develops under the posterior aspect where the stresses are concentrated (Fig. 4b).

The common denominator of these different cases of osteoarthritis presented above consists of a local increase of the articular compressive stresses. This is the mechanical cause of osteoarthritis of the knee. A logical treatment must decrease the articular pres-

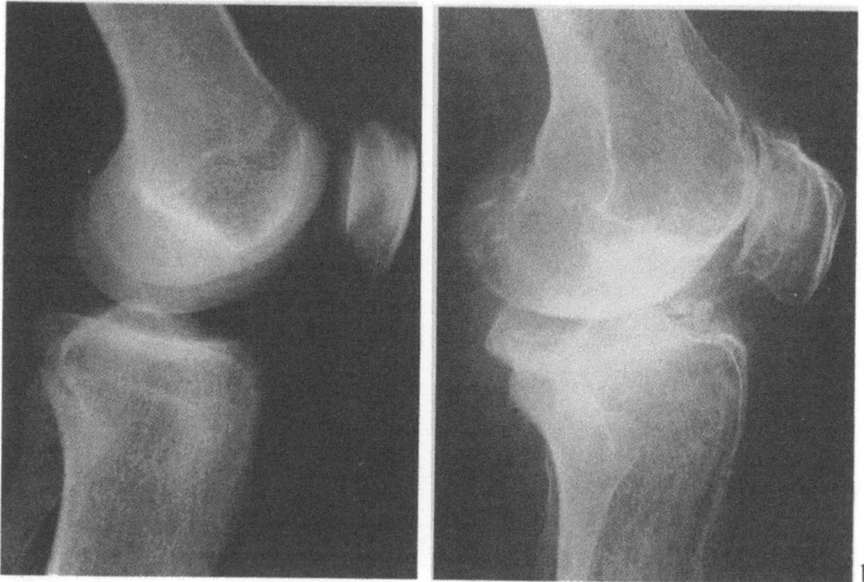

Fig. 4a, b

sure and distribute it as evenly as possible over the largest possible weight bearing surfaces. In other words, resultant R must be brought back to the centre of gravity of the articular contact surfaces. Depending on the pecularities of each particular case, this aim is attained either by an osteotomy of the upper end of the tibia, by an osteotomy of the lower end of the femur, or by correcting a deformity at a distance from the affected knee.

Understanding the mechanical situation and planning the operation requires appropriate X-rays of the patient standing with full weight on the affected knee. An A.P. X-ray of the whole limb, fully loaded, is necessary to measure accurately the deformity.

As shown by Kummer [6], the barrel vault osteotomy of the tibia which we have previously described [8, 9] represents the best choice for the treatment of medial osteoarthritis of the knee, usually associated with a varus deformity. After this operation, the articular surfaces of the tibial plateaux are perpendicular to the line of action of the resultant R. In order to bring back R to the centre of gravity of the contact surfaces, some overcorrection is necessary. Exact correction of the deformity would, in most cases, bring the knee back in the mechanical situation which caused the condition to appear and develop. Some overcorrection thus is usually necessary. In treating osteoarthritis with a varus deformity this overcorrection will bring the knee closer to the line of action of force P. Force P can then be balanced by a smaller force L (due to the weakening of the muscles) (Fig. 5).

On the A.P. X-ray of the entire lower limb under load, a line is drawn from the center of the femoral head to the mid cross section of the bone at osteotomy level, another from this point at mid cross section of the bone to the centre of the ankle (Fig. 6). The angle α formed by these two lines measures the deformity. In a normal knee angle α is equal to O. The outlines of the knee are traced on transparent paper from the A.P. X-ray of the loaded knee (Fig. 7). A half circle is drawn, concavity downwards, around the tibial tuberosi-

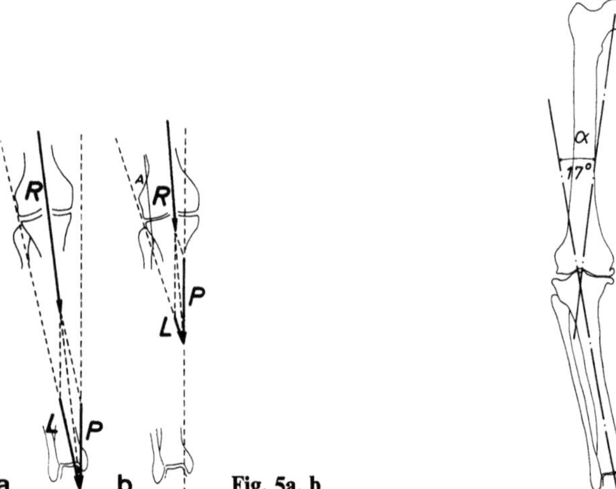

Fig. 5a, b

Fig. 6

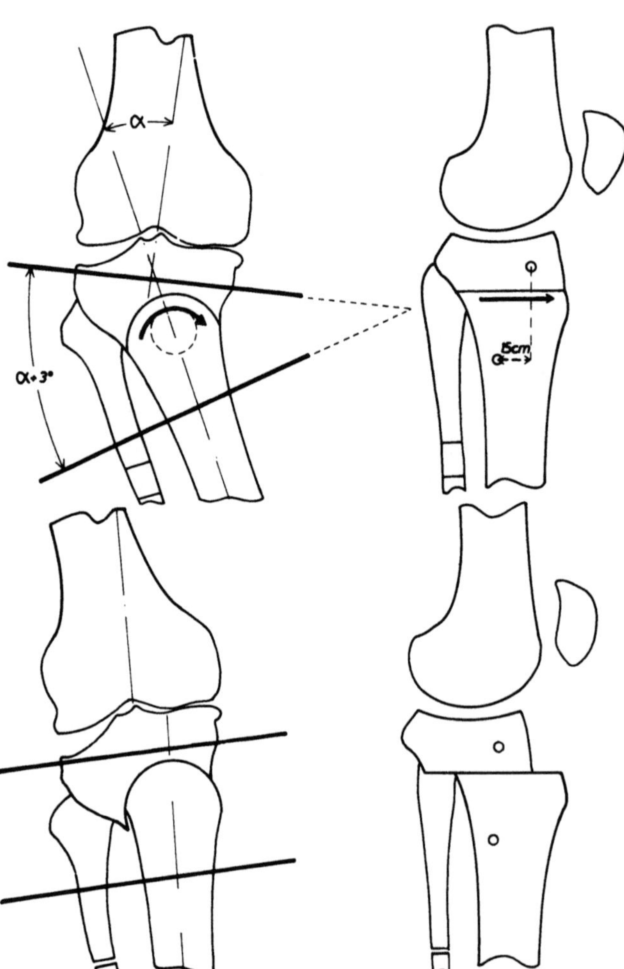

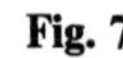

Fig. 7

ty. It corresponds to the osteotomy line. Its radius is about 2.5 cm. A transverse line is drawn through the upper diaphysis and another through the epiphysis. They form an angle $\alpha + 3°$ to $5°$. The $3°$ to $5°$ measure the desired overcorrection which will be less in a young athlete, more in an elderly obese woman. The distal fragment with its transverse line is then traced on a second transparent paper. This is then turned on the first until its transverse line runs parallel to the proximal transverse line on the first sheet of paper. The proximal fragment and the lower end of the femur are then traced on the second sheet. The operation has thus first been carried out graphically.

Barrel Vault Osteotomy – Surgical Procedure

The patient lies prone under general anaesthesia with intubation, on an operation table which is transparent to permit X-rays. No tourniquet is used in order to avoid the risks of thromboembolism.

1. If a flexion contracture exists, the skin and aponeurosis are incised longitudinally on the medial and on the lateral aspect of the knee, while the knee is flexed. These incisions give an approach to the femoral condyles. The capsule is divided transversely on the condyles using scissors. The knee is then forcefully extended, rupturing the last fibres of the posterior capsule. The aponeurosis and the skin are then sutured. This preliminary procedure is superfluous if there is no flexion contracture under anaesthesia.

2. The knee is flexed at right angle. The middle third of the fibula is approached through a postero-lateral incision between the peroneal muscles and the extensors of the toes. The periosteum is incised and carefully raised from the bone with a curved periosteal elevator. The fibula is divided obliquely with a reciprocating power saw. One should avoid tearing a fibular vein close to the medial periosteum. Bleeding from this vein may be difficult to stop.

3. The knee is extended. The tibial tuberosity is approached through a 5 cm longitudinal anterior incision and the patella tendon is dissected free. The tibia is cleaned behind the patella tendon, with a periosteal elevator. The osteotomy curve is marked by a series of holes drilled with a Kirschner wire guided by a slotted instrument introduced behind the patella tendon. The concavity of this instrument is downwards, around the tibial tuberosity.

This half circle of holes corresponds to that of the preoperative drawing. A Steinmann pin is then drilled transversely by hand through the upper third of the tibial shaft. No power drill is used to avoid heating and the subsequent muscular necrosis. The Steinmann pin is perpendicular to the axis of the shaft. A second Steinmann pin is then introduced just underneath the tibial plateaux, forming an angle $\alpha + 3°$ to $5°$ with the first pin. The angle is preset on the Pin Guide. Projected on a sagittal plane, the proximal pin lies 1 to 1.5 cm in front of the distal. The angle is controlled by X-ray. The bone is then divided along the osteotomy curve with a thin chisel. This division must be carefully carried out. One can feel the penetration of the posterior cortex by the chisel. The distal fragment is then rotated under the proximal one and brought forward until the two Steinmann pins lie parallel in the same coronal plane. Compression clamps are placed over these pins and the fragments are compressed against each other. This is done under X-ray control. The skin is closed over suction drainage.

The operation accurately achieves the desired overcorrection and also anteriorly displaces the tibial tuberosity. This further reduces compression in the femoro-tibial and patello-femoral joint.

The procedure is simple and practically bloodless. The posterior vessels gave us no problem, but the division of the bone must be carried out very carefully. A few patients have presented a postoperative palsy of the dorsi-flexors of the foot. In two of these patients, necrosis of the anterior compartment of the lower leg was found at re-exploration. Such a necrosis has no longer occurred since the distal pin is introduced by hand, avoiding the power drill. During the passage of the distal pin through the soft parts, an assistant holds the foot. If this moves, the pin is removed and inserted a little anteriorly or posteriorly. While rightening the external compression clamps, the position of the proximal fragment must be checked. This fragment can impinge into the distal one either in flexion or in recurvatum when it has been displaced too far posteriorly. An advancement of the distal fragment by 1 to 1.5 cm is recommended.

The collateral ligaments are not surgically tightened. They are not even seen. They tighten spontaneously when the mechanical disturbance which has caused them to lengthen is corrected. The collateral laxity disappears, as a rule, when the deformity has been sufficiently overcorrected.

The knee is moved actively and passively the day after surgery. The patient stands up and walks with crutches on the first or second day with progressive weight bearing on the operated knee. The Steinmann pins are removed after two months with evidence of healing on X-rays. The crutches are discarded as soon as the patient feels safe, usually two to four months after surgery.

The results of the barrel-vault osteotomy of the tibia are nearly always satisfactory if a sufficient overcorrection of the varus deformity has been achieved. Correcting the varum shortens the lever arm α of force P due to the partial body mass acting on the knee. This force P can therefore be counterbalanced by a relatively weak pull of the lateral muscles L and the resultant force R, vectorial sum of P and L, is decreased (Fig. 5). Above all, displacing the resultant R laterally redistributes the compressive stresses over larger articular weight bearing areas. Both effects of the barrel vault osteotomy overcorrecting a varus deformity diminish the intra-articular pressure. Reducing the articular compressive stresses leads to a regression of the osteoarthritic alterations which can be read on the X-rays.

The 65-year-old patient (Fig. 8a–d) presented severe osteoarthritis of both knees with a varus deformity. The increase of the subchondral sclerosis under the medial tibial plateax substantiates the localized concentration of stress. Similarly, a dense triangle can be seen under the posterior aspect of the articular surfaces on the lateral X-ray. The correction attained was 26° for the right knee, 34° for the left. After the barrel-vault osteotomies which overcorrected the deformities, the subchondral sclerosis regresses under the medial plateaux whereas the subchondral sclerosis and the cancellous structure appear more pronounced under the lateral plateaux. The dense triangle has disappeared. A normal joint space has developed. The follow-up is 6 years for the right knee, 7 years for the left. The clinical result is excellent.

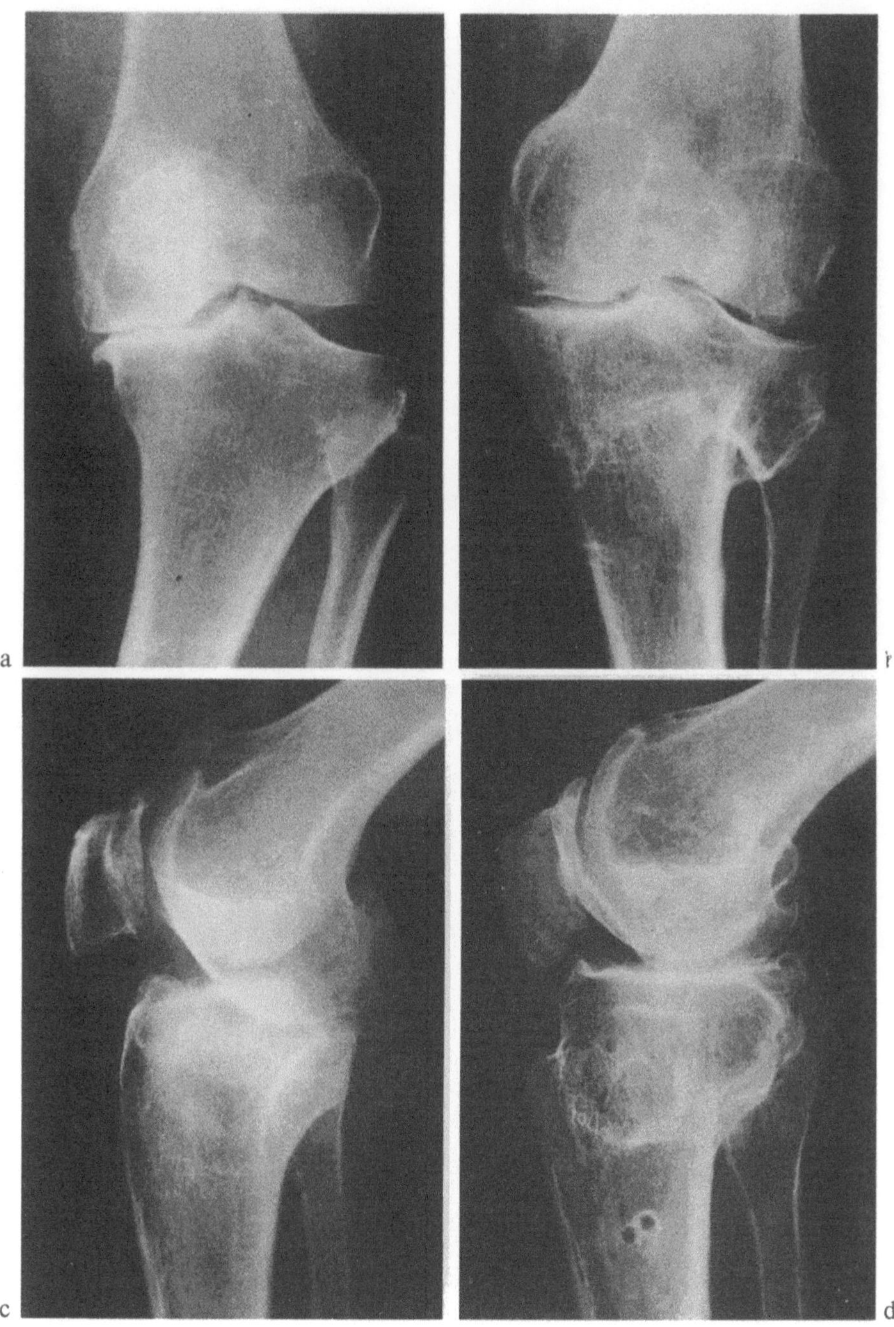

Fig. 8a–d

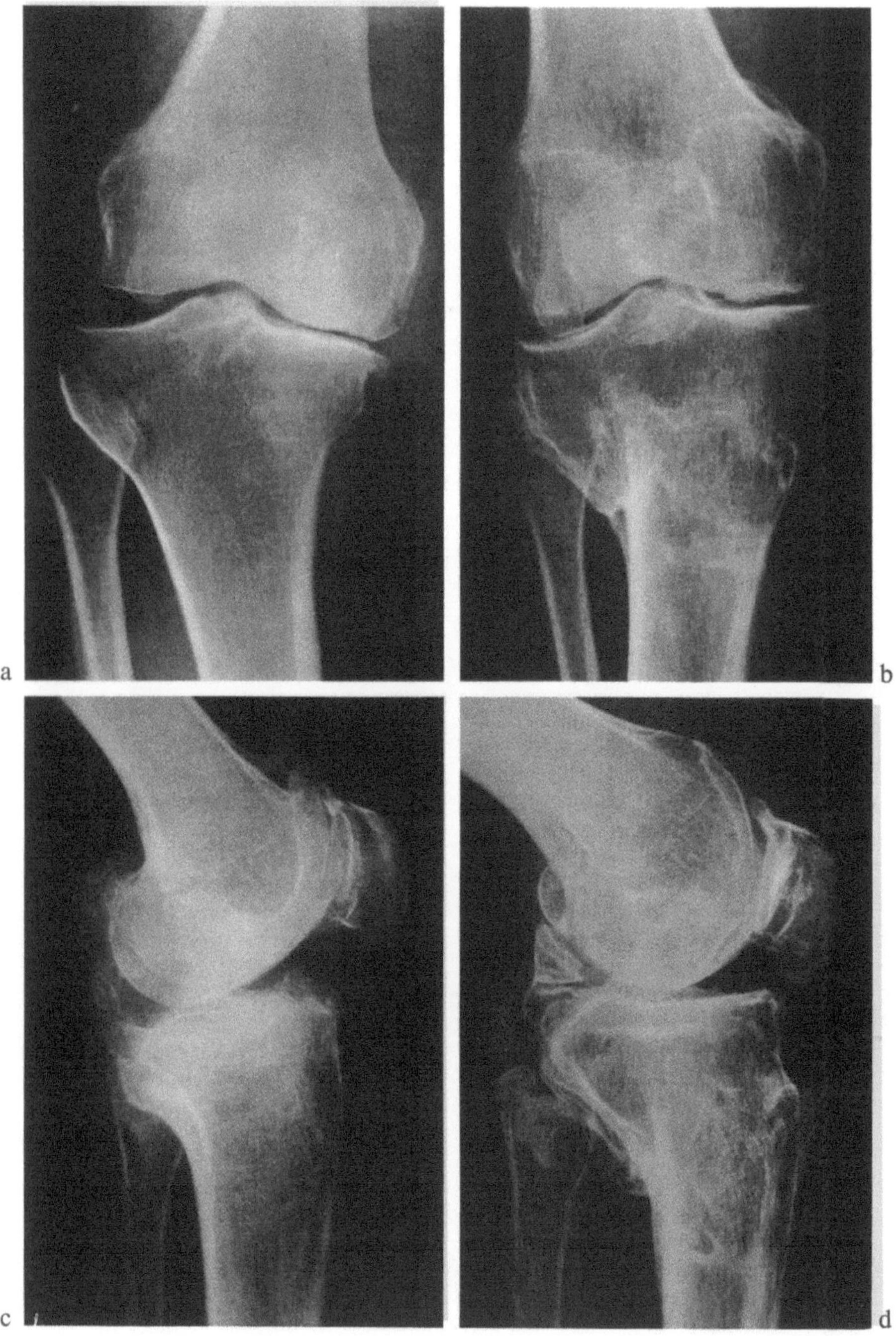

Fig. 9a–d

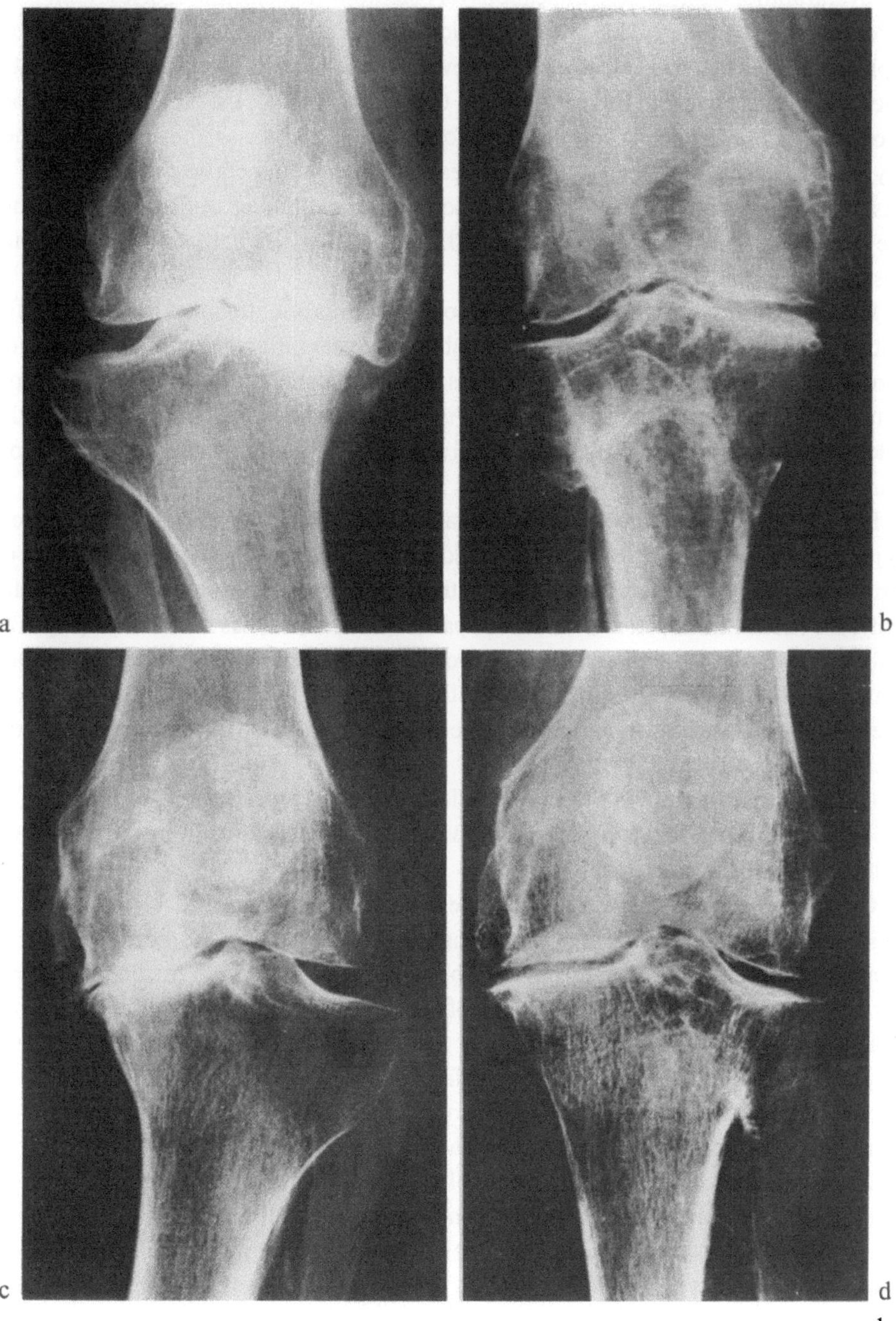

Fig. 10a–d

Several authors restrict their indications for osteotomy to deformities of less than 15° to 20°, some even to less than 10°, without flexion contracture. Beyond that, they propose to replace the knee by a total prosthesis. However, on one hand, the long term results of the knee prostheses appear to be very dubious. On the other hand, the procedure described above allows to overcorrect very severe deformities. In such cases, the results are generally good to excellent, after a simple and nearly bloodless procedure. Subluxation of an unstable knee has not been a contraindication for this method, in our experience. When the deformity is sufficiently overcorrected, the ligaments tighten spontaneously and ensure the stability of the joint.

The 75-year-old patient (Fig. 9) presents osteoarthritis of both knees with varus deformities. Both joints are subluxated and unstable. Five years after overcorrection of the deformities, the laxity has disappeared. The sclerotic triangle under the medial tibial plateau has regressed and the lateral plateau is now underlined by a normal subchondral sclerosis. This demonstrates that the lateral aspect of the joint now takes part in the load transmission (Fig. 9b).

Far reaching destruction of the medial plateau does not hinder recovery of a satisfactory joint function. The knee of the 62-year-old female patient (Fig. 10a) presents such a destruction. Eight years after a barrel-vault osteotomy of the tibia overcorrecting the deformity, the medial tibial plateau which was partially destroyed, has remodelled (Fig. 10b). Subchondral sclerosis and cancellous structure are practically symmetrical under both plateaux. This demonstrates an optimal distribution and a reduction of the articular compressive stresses. Meanwhile, the other knee has been operated on with a similarly good result (Fig. 10c, d).

Old age does not seem to be a contraindication for this procedure. The capacity of the living tissues to regenerate persists until the end of life. This is demonstrated by the results achieved in patients over 80.

Osteoarthritis with a valgus deformity presents a problem more difficult to solve. A valgus knee is closer to the line of action of force P. This could entail some mechanical advantage. Correction of the deformity will bring the knee away from the line of action of force P, thus lengthening the lever arm a of force P. The moment Pa must be adapted to the abnormally great force L in such a way that the resultant R comes to act at the centre of gravity of the femoro-tibial contact surfaces. This increases the load R supported by the knee. Therefore, the reduction of the articular pressure cannot be achieved through a diminution of the load but only through an increase of the weight-bearing surfaces.

In a normal knee, R acts at the centre of gravity of the articular contact surfaces, perpendicular to the latter. The valgus deformity changes the direction of the femur and of the muscles L in relation to the line of action of force P. Hereby, the resultant R becomes more oblique and is displaced laterally. It comes to act obliquely in relation to the plane tangential to the tibial plateaux. It acts on this plane with a perpendicular component M and a transverse component T (Fig 11a). The obliquity of resultant R explains why the compressive stresses are increased and concentrated in the vicinity of the intercondylar eminence rather than on the margin of the lateral plateau. This is made obvious by the subchondral sclerosis delineated by a convex outline (Fig 3). There exists thus an essential difference from osteoarthritis with a varus deformity.

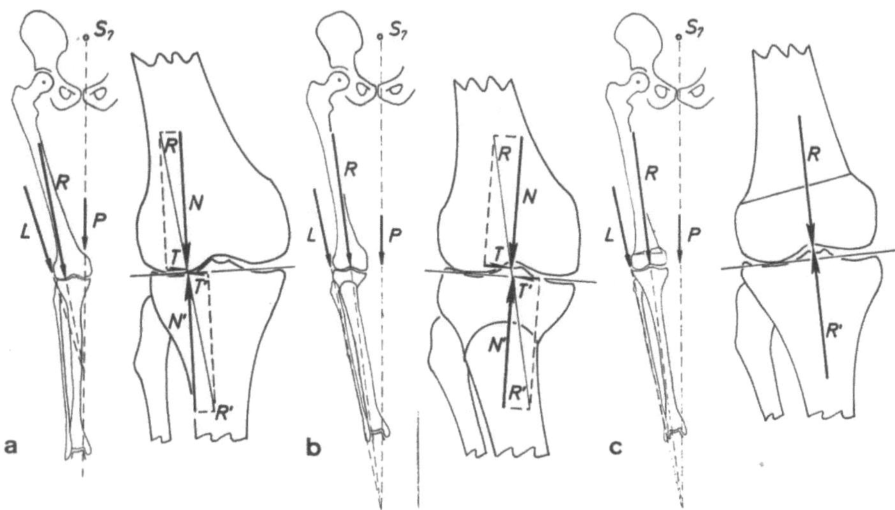

Fig. 11a–c

An osteotomy correcting the deformity will change the orientation of the femur and of the muscles L, bringing the intersection of forces P and L away from the knee.

If the overcorrection is attained through a barrel vault osteotomy of the tibia (Fig 11b), the upper end of the latter turns as does force R. This keeps acting obliquely on the plane tangential to the tibial plateaux. The compressive stresses must remain concentrated close to the intercondylar eminence and cannot be transmitted through the medial plateau which is too oblique. Moreover, correcting the valgus deformity without moving force R medially lengthens the leverarm α of force P. Equilibrium requires a greater force L and the resultant R is increased. This explains the poor results following a high tibial osteotomy used correct a valgus deformity.

When the valgus deformity is corrected through an osteotomy of the lower end of the femur (Fig 11c), the knee turns in a direction opposite that of the resultant force R. Hence, force R comes to act perpendicularly to the plane tangential to the tibial plateau and the stresses can be evenly distributed.

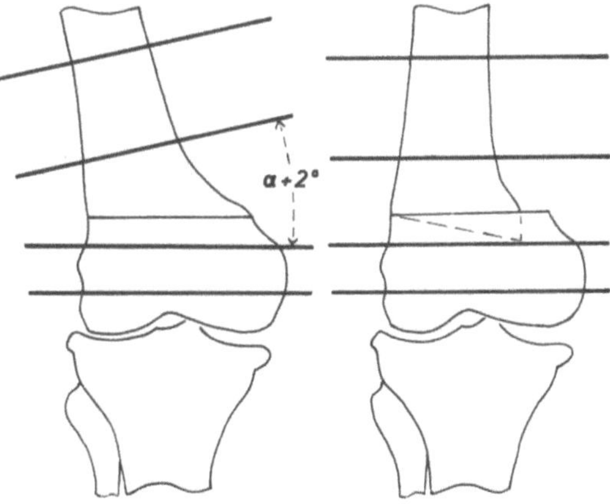

Fig. 12

A long X-ray showing the whole limb is used in order to measure the deformity. A line is drawn from the centre of the femoral head to the mid cross section of the femur at osteotomy level, just proximal to the condyles. Another line is drawn from this point to the centre of the ankle. The angle α which they form measures the deformity.

The outlines of the joint are traced on transparent paper from the A.P. X-ray in standing (Fig 12). The osteotomy will be carried out transversely proximal to the condyles. Two transverse lines are drawn through the condyles, parallel to each other. Two more transverse lines are drawn through the distal part of the femoral shaft. They form with the former and angle $\alpha + 1°$ to $2°$. These $1°$ to $2°$ provide the overcorrection which should avoid replacing the knee in the mechanical conditions under which osteoarthritis appeared and developed. The distal fragment and the tibia with its transverse lines is then traced on a second sheet of transparent paper which is rotated on the first until the four transverse lines, those through the condyles and those through the shaft, are made parallel. The proximal fragment is finally traced on the second sheet of transparent paper in this position. Again the surgical procedure thus has been carried out graphically.

Osteoarthritis with a valgus deformity does not usually present any flexion contracture. Posterior capsulotomy is thus rarely indicated.

Distal Femoral Osteotomy — Surgical Procedure

The patient is under general anaesthesia with intubation. He lies prone on a table transparent to X-rays, a folded drape under the knee. The supracondylar region is approached medially through a 5 cm longitudinal incision, between the vastus medialis and the intermuscular septum. The periosteum is raised from the bone anteriorly and posteriorly. The periosteal elevator is left behind the supracondylar region to protect the popliteal vessels. Two parallel Steinmann pins are inserted transversely through the condyles, using the pin insertion guide. The distal one lies as close to the joint space as possible but should not penetrate the joint. Two other parallel pins are inserted through the shaft. The form with the two former an angle $\alpha + 1°$ to $2°$ ensured by the pin insertion guide. The most distal and the most proximal pins are inserted through short separate incisions, the others through the surgical wound.

The femur is divided supracondylarly with a reciprocating saw and, eventually, a thin chisel, keeping part of the lateral cortex intact. After the medial, anterior and posterior aspects of the proximal fragment are levelled, the latter is impinged into the distal using the lateral cortex as a hinge, until the four Steinmann pins lie parallel to each other in the same coronal plane. Two compression clamps, each equipped with four mobile units, are adapted to the Steinmann pins and the fragments are fixed under compression. The aponeurosis and the skin are sutured over suction drainage.

As after the barrel-vault osteotomy, the patient moves the knee the day following surgery. He stands up and walks with partial weight bearing from the second day. Two crutches are used during the first weeks. The nails are removed after two months and evidence of union. They may hinder somewhat the flexion of the knee which soon becomes freely mobile after their removal.

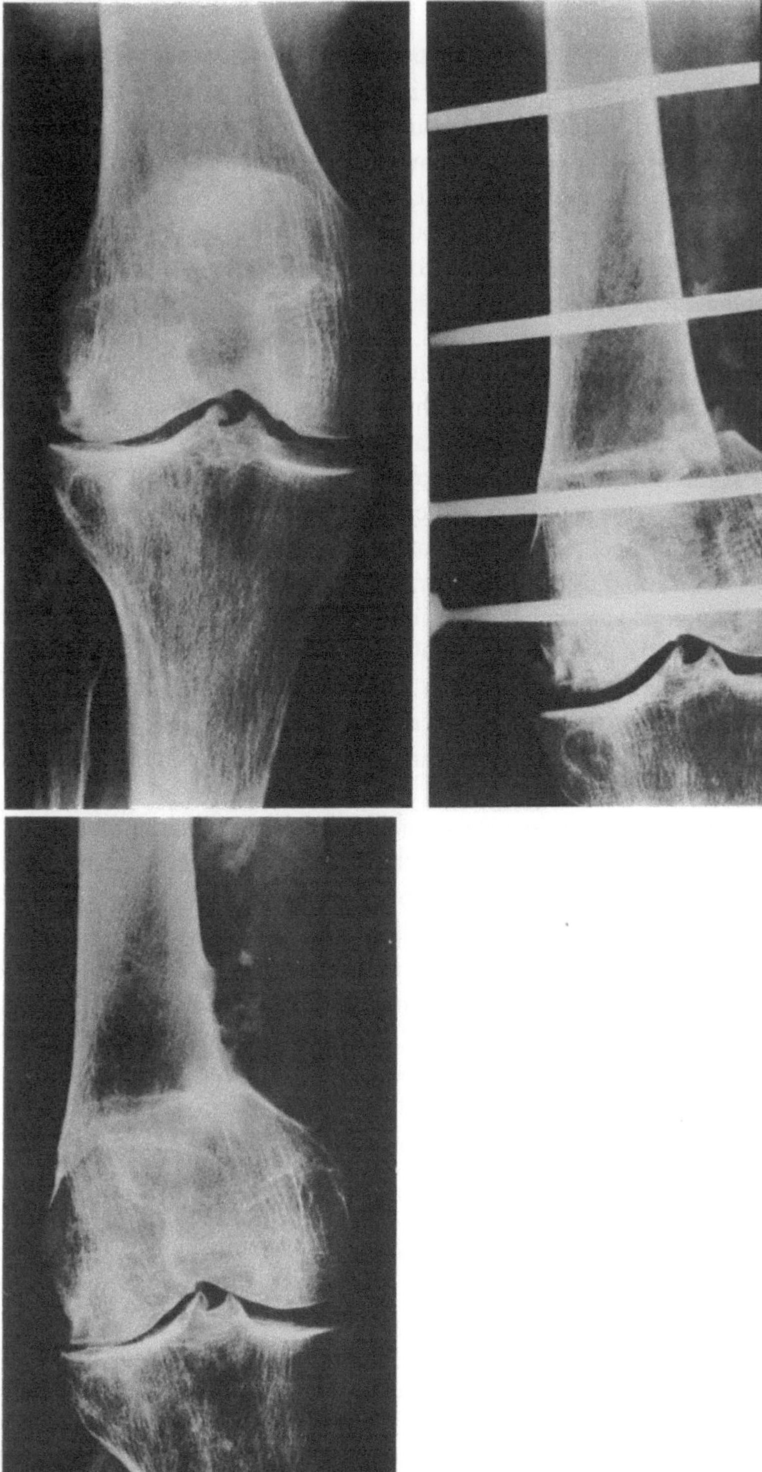

Fig. 13

The 74-year-old female patient (Fig 13) presents a severe osteoarthritis of the knee with a valgus deformity. The subchondral sclerosis is increased under the lateral plateau, the subchondral sclerosis and the cancellous structure have faded away under the medial plateau. The X-ray immediately after surgery shows the penetration of the proximal fragment into the distal and the position of the pins. Later, the subchondral sclerosis and the cancellous structure tend to become symmetrical under the medial and lateral plateaux. This substantiates an even distribution of the compressive stresses in the joint.

There is yet another method of recentring the load and of distributing the compressive stresses over the largest weight bearing surfaces, in some cases of osteoarthritis. It consists in correcting a deformity at a distance from the affected knee. This deformity is probably the first cause of the condition. However, this approach of the problem lies beyond the limits of the present work and has been dealt with elsewhere [8, 9].

The results of 125 tibial and femoral osteotomies followed from 1 to 12 years confirm our theory [9]. Dividing the bone is not sufficient to ensure a favourable evolution. A good result depends on a proper redistribution of the stresses which usually can only be achieved by an overcorrection of the deformity.

Restitution of the normal alignement of the femur and the tibia without overcorrection in 18 cases gives only 10 satisfactory results. When the deformity is not corrected or is undercorrected, the results are poor or just fair (7 out of 7 cases). Only a sufficient overcorrection gives 101 excellent and good results among 111 cases.

A detailed analysis of the results of surgery carried out for such cases is in preparation progress.

The proposed surgical procedures require accurate graphical planning and precise surgery. However the sources of error in measuring the deformity when the latter is servere and when there exists a collateral laxity with instability of the joint. In planning the operation, these factors must be taken into account [9].

In some severe cases, surgery resulted in an exaggerated overcorrection. In these cases, regression of the signs of osteoarthritis seemed to be much quicker and led to the reappearance of a large joint space. Two patients were reoperated on because they felt impeded by the postoperative deformity although they were painfree. Their overcorrection was reduced to a reasonable degree. We had the opportunity to reoperate on a patient who had undergone surgery elsewhere for a varus deformity. She presented a 25° valgum. We reduced the overcorrection to 2°.

The reoperation should be carried out in the old operative site: high tibial osteotomy to reduce the valgum deformity resulting from exaggerated overcorrection of a varus deformity: low femoral osteotomy to reduce the varus deformity resulting from exaggerated overcorrection of a valgus knee through a femoral osteotomy.

The diminution and even distribution of the compressive stresses in the joints result in a return to normal of the structure of the bone under the tibial plateau. A large joint space reappears in the X-ray of the loaded knee. This implies the development of tissue in the joint. It seemed interesting to investigate the tissue growing in a joint space subjected again to stresses probably of physiological magnitude. To this aim, Fujisawa et al. [3] carried out arthroscopies in a series of knees before and months or years after a high tibial osteotomy for osteoarthritis. They took biopsies of the newly developed tissue. Before surgery, the articular surfaces in the osteoarthritic region consisted of eburnated bone.

Two years after a sufficient overcorrection of a varus deformity through a high tibial osteotomy, the articular surfaces of the weight bearing area appear covered by a tissue similar to hyaline cartilage. Histological examination shows fibrocartilage the deep layers of which appear to remodel into hyaline cartilage. This evolution demonstrates the amazing capacity of regeneration of the skeletal tissues when subjected to mechanical stresses of physiological quality and magnitude. Such a capacity of regeneration should make orthopaedic surgeons reluctant to use prostheses in the treatment of osteoarthritis. There exists a possibility for the osteoarthritic alterations to regress. This is equivalent to a biological healing.

References

1. Blaimont P, Burnotte J, Baillon JM, Duby P (1971) Contribution biomécanique à l'étude des conditions d'équilibre dans le genou normal et pathologique. Acta Orthop Belg 37, 573-591
2. Coventry MB (1973) Osteotomy about the knee for degenerative and rheumatoid arthritis. Indications, operative technique and results. J Bone Jt Surg A 55:23-48
3. Fujisawa Y, Matsumoto N, Takakura Y, Mii Y, Shiomi S, Masuhara K (1976) The effect of high tibial osteotomy on osteoarthritis of the knee. An arthroscopical study of 26 knee joints. Clin Orthop Surg (Jap) 11:576-590
4. Insall J, Shoji H, Mayer V (1974) High tibial osteotomy. J Bone Jt Surg 56 A:1397-1405
5. Jackson JP, Waugh W, Green JP (1969) High tibial osteotomy for osteoarthritis of the knee. J Bone Jt Surg 51 B:88-94
6. Kummer B (1977) Biomechanische Grundlagen „beanspruchungsändernder" Osteotomien im Bereich des Kniegelenks. Z Orthop 19:923-928
7. MacIntosh DL, Welsh RP (1977) Joint debridement. A complement to high tibial osteotomy in the treatment of degenerative arthritis of the knee. J Bone Jt Surg 59 A:1094-1097 (1977)
8. Maquet P (1970) Biomechanics and osteoarthritis of the knee. S.I.C.O.T. XIe Congrès, Mexico, 1969. Imprimerie des Sciences, Bruxelles, pp. 317-357
9. Maquet P (1977) Biomechanics of the knee. Berlin Heidelberg New York: Springer 1976. Franz. Übers.: Biomécanique du genou. Springer: Berlin, Heidelberg, New York
10. Pauwels F (1973b) Kurzer Überblick über die mechanische Beanspruchung des Knochens und ihre Bedeutung für die funktionelle Anpassung. Z Orthop 111:681-705

Translation from the German: Maquet P (1979) Korrekturosteotomien in der Behandlung der Kniearthrose. Orthopäde 8:296-308 © Springer Verlag 1979

Principles of Corrective Osteotomies in Osteoarthrosis of the Knee

H. Wagner*

Joint deformities and axial malalignment play a much more important role in the lower extremity than in the upper extremity due to the fact that the lower limbs are weight bearing extremities. This is the reason why femoral and tibial deformities result to a greater extent in abnormal wear of their respective joints. Consequently, these deformities contribute in a much greater degree to the development of secondary osteoarthritis and its sequelae. These facts have to be considered when contemplating the indication for corrective surgery as well as when considering the quality of the surgery.

The accurate evaluation of the deformities, not only in respect to their morphological aspect but also in their influence on function, provides the basis on which to formulate a plan of therapy. Drawings are made from the radiographs which serve as models for the corrective osteotomies. One should always utilize these drawings when dealing with realignment osteotomies. To plan and execute surgical correction using only standing radiographs which demonstrate the effect of weight bearing without analyzing the function of the extremity is inadequate. One should always consider the basic rule that we treat patients and not x-rays.

Radiographs are, however, an important part of the evaluation of the patient and should always completely demonstrate the deformity. Different locations and varied forms of the different types of classical deformities may require special radiographic views (Hafner and Meuli). The examination of joint motion under fluoroscopic image intensification can be very instructive. This is possible without significant irradition if the image intensifier is equipped with a video memory unit. To demonstrate the actual amount of a deformity, it is important to bring the plane of the deformity parallel to that of the x-ray film. As an example, in an anterolateral axis deviation of a long bone, i.e. a bone with varus deformation and anterior bowing, the deformity will be demonstrated in the standard anteroposterior and lateral projections to a lesser degree than that actually present. Only when the plane of deformity is parallel to the x-ray film is the full amount of angulation recognizable. In the above example, this means that the anteroposterior view should be taken with the leg externally rotated.

---

* Orthopädische Klinik Wichernhaus, Surgeon-in-Chief: Prof. Dr. Heinz Wagner, D-8503 Alt-dorf/Nürnberg, Federal Republic of Germany

These special radiographic views are then used as the basis for drawings in which the osteotomies can be simulated. In realignment osteotomies which influence the length of an extremity, the magnification factor of the radiographs must be considered and is usually estimated to be approximately 20 percent. If there is any doubt as to the degree of magnification, an object of known dimensions can be placed alongside the extremity in the plane of the joint and projected onto the film. It can then be measured on the film to determine the amount of magnification.

An important question with far reaching consequences is to determine to what extent the soft tissues contribute to the functional limitation of motion. This limitation is primarily the result of the bony deformity. If the distal femur is angulated in a flexed position from the proximal segment, this results in a loss of extension of the knee joint. This can in time cause a contracture of the posterior joint capsule and further increase the knee flexion contracture. A supracondylar osteotomy to gain full extension would require an overcorrection of the bony deformity in the distal femur to compensate for the soft tissue contracture. However, when this patient begins to bear weight in extension, the posterior capsule is put under tension and will stretch so that the knee will develope a recurvatum deformity with the passage of time. To avoid this problem, the soft tissue contracture has to be eliminated preoperatively through the use of range of motion exercises and positional splinting. Only after the contracture has been eliminated should an osteotomy be performed.

Different principles apply in knees which have lost extension secondary to degenerative arthritis. The benefit of an osteotomy achieving full extension would be lost in two or three weeks in an arthritic patient because of the recurrence of the flexion deformity. In degenerative arthritis of the knee, experience has shown that overcorrection with ten degrees of recurvatum has to be obtained to achieve a long lasting good result with maintenance of full extension.

A special problem is the evaluation of deformities and the formulation of a treatment plan in a lower extremity with its multiple neighboring joints whose functions influence each other. The correct sequence of corrective procedures is of great importance. Close cooperation between surgeon and physiotherapist has to be coordinated to avoid unnecessary therapeutic steps.

A good example of this is the residual of poliomyelitis with peripherally progressive involvement. These patients frequently present with hip flexion contractures, flexion and valgus deformities of the knee, an equinus contracture of the ankle joint, and a valgus instability of the paralytic foot. On superficial inspection, these deformities give the impression that operative correction at all three joint levels would be required. In reality, the primary problem of these patients is the paralysis of the muscles below the knee and a partial paralysis of the thigh muscles. The contractures about the hip, knee, and ankle joints are the result of positioning during the acute phase of poliomyelitis and resultant muscle imbalances. These contractures cause the patient to become nonambulatory in spite of the fact that the remaining musculature has the potential to stabilize the limb. The minimal use of the extremity has resulted in disuse atrophy of the musculature which mimics a much more severe form of paralysis.

In such poliomyelitis cases, it is mandatory to preoperatively evaluate the extent of improvement to be expected from physiotherapy on the strength of the innervated muscle and to what extent splinting can relieve acquired joint contractures. Only after careful and consistent physical therapy can one make these determinations. It is advisable to provide temporary stability to the extremity during this evaluation period by the use of simple lightweight braces. This can often be accomplished through the use of plaster or plastic splints.

An incompetent m. triceps surae associated with a knee flexion contracture results in an unstable knee. This can be effectively overcome with the use of a below-knee orthosis with the walking heel positioned slightly more forward than usual on the sole. The potential for rehabilitation of the musculature under physiotherapy, especially after restoration of ambulation, is remarkable. In addition, joint contractures improve under this intense physiotherapy so that functional stability is frequently achieved solely by stabilizing the foot in a slight equinus position. Occasionally, supracondylar osteotomy of the femur is additionally required to achieve this goal of stability.

In the absence of paralysis, preoperative physical therapy is important for many reasons prior to corrective osteotomies. Patients must learn how to use their Lofstrand crutches and how to walk with a partial weight-bearing gait pattern on the involved extremity. This is practiced with the use of a bathroom scale. Isometric muscle tightening exercises not only improve the patient's strength but also improve the quality of the soft tissue in the area of the proposed surgical incision. The patients are familiarized with the active assisted range of motion exercises that will be begun after surgery. All of these things greatly facilitate the postoperative physical therapy program.

The personality of the patient has to be considered along with all of his domestic and professional problems when deciding upon the indications for a corrective osteotomy. The patient should have a reasonable understanding of the basic treatment principles and demonstrate the proper motivation. These are the prerequisites for cooperation with the treatment plan and physiotherapy. Osteotomies which are done primarily prophylactically to avoid the development of future problems require that the patients have insight into the natural history of their disease. It requires special confidence in the physician to submit to surgical treatment before onset of any complaints.

In osteoarthritis of the knee joint, the primary pathology is progressive wear of the damaged, degenerated hyaline joint cartilage followed by intraarticular disturbance of joint motion. However, in the majority of patients, the clinical picture demonstrates significant malalignment and ligamentous instability.

During the time of growth, the planes of weight bearing joint surfaces are influenced by the alternating forces generated by the passive osseous and ligamentous structures on one side and the active muscles of the other side. This results in an alignment which causes a maximum of compression forces and a minimum of shear forces on the joint surfaces. The optimal axial alignment varies with constitutional characteristics such as body proportions and muscle power. Females with weaker musculature as well as patients with muscle paralysis develop a mild valgus position as their optimal knee alignment. Males and very athletic females who have a stronger musculature develop a mild varus position of their knees. Racial differences are also noted.

For the orthopaedic surgeon it is a very common experience to follow knee joints with advanced arthritic changes on x-ray for several years while the patient has minimal symptoms and remains active and employable. Painful decompensation frequently occurs

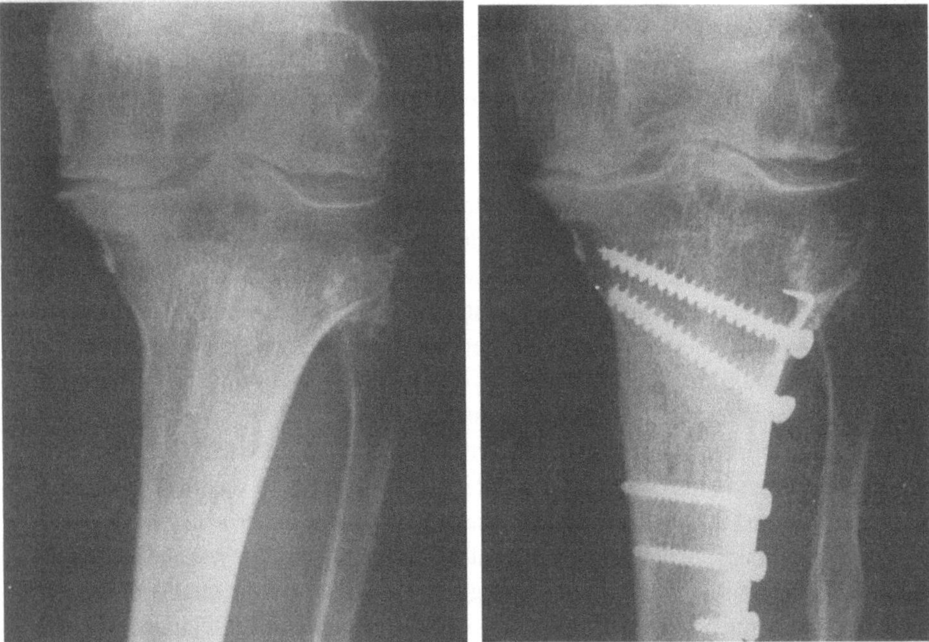

Fig. 1. A Osteoarthritis of the right knee in a 62 year old male with a varus deformity and narrowing of the medial joint space. **B** Two years after proximal tibial osteotomy demonstrating widening of the articular joint space and remodeling of the subchondral bone

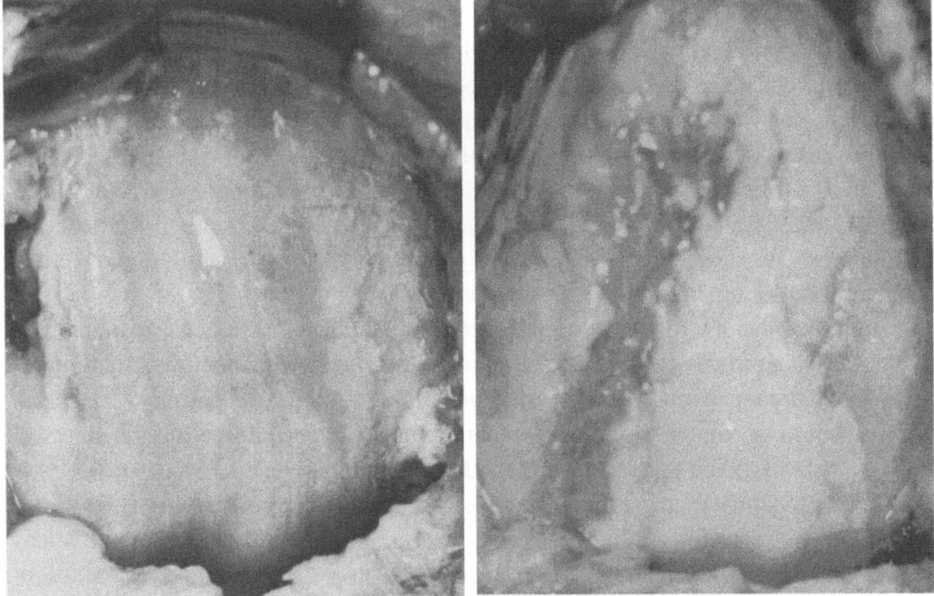

Fig. 2. Intraoperative photographs of the patient whose radiographs are shown in Figure 1. **A** Eburnated bony surface of the medial femoral condyle at the time of proximal tibial osteotomy. **B** The same femoral condyle two years later on the occasion of hardware removal showing fibrocartilaginous tissue formation following realignment osteotomy of the proximal tibia

rather suddenly when the stable tracking of the joint is lost due to malalignment of the bones, laxity of the ligamentous structures, and atrophy of the musculature.

Malalignment of the arthritic knee is typically caused by the asymmetrical wear of the joint cartilage damaged by systemic or traumatic insults, or a long period of continuous abuse. Through the loss of cartilaginous tissue, the radiological joint space narrows. The bony ends of the femur and tibia approach each other and cause an axial malalignment of the extremity with the affected compartment lying on the concave side of the limb.

Continuous asymmetrical loss of cartilage height leads to an increase in the axial deformity. Symmetrical joint loading with even pressure distribution over the entire joint surface is therefore no longer possible. Asymmetrical loading results in high concentration of pressure forces over a small surface area. The compression forces are increased over the concave side of the deformity. This leads to an increase in wear and, subsequently, to a progression of the angulation. In addition, the ligamentous structures become lax and incompetent. The joint structures on the convex side are subjected to tensile forces during loading. This leads to overstretching of the ligamentous structures. The combination of the ligamentous laxity on the concave side and elongation on the convex side leads to compromized ligamentous stability of the knee.

Lack of muscle use results in atrophy which causes the arthritic knee joints to become progressively more unstable. This in itself is a more significant factor in limiting ambulation than the arthritic changes of the joint surfaces. In almost all forms of arthritis, the knee tends to assume a slightly flexed position for protection and comfort, and this results in synovial scarring and osteophyte formation. All of these factors limit knee extension and eventually result in a fixed contracture of the posterior capsule.

The malalignment in degenerative arthritis of the knee joint becomes an independent biomechanical factor. Together with other structural and functional causes, it contributes to the progression of the arthritis. Surgical correction of the malalignment therefore eliminates an important etiologic factor for the progressive joint destruction. At the same time, the realignment improves the biomechanical response to the stress of loading. The corrective osteotomy frequently causes a dramatic improvement of symptoms caused by malalignment. This impressively proves that malalignment and abnormal loading are important etiologic factors for the development of pain.

Improved function allows the arthritic joint to recover structurally. The circumscribed sclerosis close to the joint surface is replaced by more homogeneous cancellous bone. Fibrocartilaginous regeneration eventually covers the eburnated bony surface (Fig. 1 and 2).

Indications

The purposes of corrective osteotomy are to remove the intraarticular causes of loss of motion, to improve and stabilize ligamentous instability, and to strengthen the musculature. Improved functional use of the extremity is the most important factor in allowing the arthritic knee to recover. The closer one comes to recreating normal biomechanical conditions, the better the prognosis for the joint. When dealing with complex deformities which might require multiple osteotomies, the degree of improvement one can achieve must be balanced against the surgical effort to accomplish this goal. This decision demands experience and requires the consideration of many aspects: (1) the patient's age and life expectancy, (2) the severity of the arthritic involvement and degree of malalignment, and (3) the patient's job-related and recreational/physical requirements. One must also consider whether these corrective osteotomies, desirable as they might be, can be realistically accomplished. The surgeon has to realistically evaluate his own technical expertise and the facilities available to him. The soft tissues, quality of bone, and type and location of the deformity must be thoroughly considered in determining the degree of difficulty in each individual case.

In a younger patient with strong healthy bone structures and a long life expectancy, complex osteotomies might be desirable, and the young patient can be expected to better tolerate extensive surgical procedures. In an older patient, perfect correction is more difficult to achieve secondary to osteoporosis. The long term prognostic outlook is of lesser importance while early rehabilitation to an independent functional status is of prime importance. Therefore, a partical correction requiring a minor procedure might be a desirable compromise in the older patient.

The amount of deformity at which surgical correction becomes necessary varies with the age of the patient. In general, one can expect that a flexion contracture of more than five degrees and an axial deviation in the frontal plane of greater than 10° will cause or accelerate the development of degenerative arthritis. When these conditions are present correction by surgical means is therefore indicated.

The optimal timing of surgery is an important consideration in corrective osteotomies. In older patients, osteotomies are not usually performed to improve long term prognosis. The goal in these patients is the immediate improvement of function. This is achieved by arresting the progression of the already advanced arthritis with improvement of stability and reduction of pain. One must consider the fact that arthritis in older patients does not run a continuously progressive course but tends to have periodic exacerbations. Stationary phases without progression of clinical or radiological findings sometimes last for decades. In spite of advanced arthritic changes and loss of motion, these patients are functional and without complaints. It is not advisable to perform a corrective osteotomy during one of these stationary phases since the patients condition will not usually improve. An exception is a severe malalignment or functional disability which may demand surgical treatment during any phase of their course. The optimal time to perform a corrective osteotomy is when radiological findings, deformity, instability, and subjective complaints show progression. A greater psychological gain is obtained by an operation at this time because the patient feels subjective improvement. This psychological advantage can not be routinely predicted when surgery is performed during the stationary phase.

A posttraumatic axial malalignment which requires surgical correction should be treated as early as possible to avoid the development of posttraumatic arthritis. Early osteotomies are indicated for axial malunions of femoral and tibial fractures and also for isolated traumatic insults to the joint surface where these osteotomies provide relief from abnormal axial weight bearing on the involved area.

Stabilization by means of internal fixation has a decisive advantage in performing corrective osteotomies about the knee. A stable osteosynthesis is the only means by which exact correction can be achieved and maintained long enough to allow bony union. It is also the only method which will allow range of motion exercises and limited functional use of the extremity immediately following reconstruction of physiologic and anatomic conditions. This type of postoperative management avoids immobilization and therefore prevents the complications of stiffness and further limitations of motion inherent in any immobilization. In the aged, the stable osteotomy might enhance the patients survival by allowing rapid return to function and avoiding strict bedrest. Early range of motion exercises are a fundamental prerequisite for the structural rehabilitation of an arthritic knee. They contribute to the formation of a new fibrocartilaginous coverage of the joint surfaces. Another important advantage of stable osteosynthesis is the fact that corrective osteotomies can be performed in close proximity to the joint surface while retaining firm fixation of the short fragment.

Corrective osteotomies in degenerative arthritis of the knee are technically demanding procedures which require a great deal of experience. One technical problem relates to the osteoporotic bone which is frequently encountered due to a recent decrease in activity level or secondary to advanced age. This requires very careful fixation by osteosynthesis devices and a very exacting fit of the osteotomy surfaces. This is the only means to achieve sufficient stability in osteoporotic bone. Another technical problem arises from the fact that surgery is performed on a recumbent patient while the corrected extremity has to be functional when the patient is weight bearing in an upright position. Specifically, the correction of a knee flexion contracture requires correction in the recumbent position in order to maintain full extension of the knee until full weight bearing can be resumed six to eight weeks postoperatively. The correction of a knee flexion contracture of greater than five degrees should usually be performed in the supracondylar area. An osteotomy through the proximal tibia necessarily results in posterior displacement of the distal tibial segment. This can result in a situation where bone healing may be delayed because of the bending forces that act through the osteotomy site. In addition, the tibial osteotomy results in a forward inclination of the tibial plateau and creates shear forces within the joint under physiologic loading. When correcting a flexion contracture by means of a supracondylar osteotomy, an overcorrection to create 10° of recurvatum is necessary. If this overcorrection is not achieved, the flexion contracture will recur within the first few postoperative days. Experience has shown that this overcorrection facilitates postoperative physical therapy. Full extension is obtained three weeks after surgery and usually persists for a long period of time.

Another important consideration in performing corrective osteotomies is the ligamentous laxity. If at all possible, this should be corrected during the same procedure to prevent the conversion of a medial instability, for instance, into a lateral instability after the corrective osteotomy. One way to achieve this with minimal effort and a reliable effect is to remove the bony insertion of the ligament with a thin wafer of bone and reattach it under tension.

The correct choice of osteosynthesis devices is also important. External fixation using Steinman pins and an external compression apparatus is easier to use especially for the inexperienced surgeon. It allows the opportunity for postoperative adjustment of the correction whenever the position is unsatisfactory. The surgical procedure is of lesser magnitude because the exposure can be limited to the osteotomy site. Further exposure necessary to allow implantation of internal fixation devices is therefore eliminated. A significant disadvantage of external fixation is less stable fixation which is especially important in epiphyseal osteotomies close to joints and in atrophic, osteoporotic bones. A second disadvantage is the bulky and cumbersome external compression apparatus. These disadvantages preclude the use of external fixation in older patients.

Internal fixation with stable osteosynthesis is doubtlessly a more elegant procedure. It achieves functional stability of the osteotomy by use of implantable devices that do not interfere with postoperative physical therapy and ambulation. The patient becomes independent of care earlier and hospitalization time is therefore shortened. Even in osteotomies very close to the joint surface, internal fixation assures reliable stability. Such a stable osteosynthesis is technically much more demanding and has a greater risk of infection because of the retained foreign material. This form of treatment therefore requires optimal surgical facilities.

Next to the technically demanding execution and stabilization of the corrective osteotomy, the postoperative physical therapy is of prime importance. Preoperative institution of the exercise program by the physiotherapist has proven to be of great benefit. Immediately after the operation the exercises are easily continued. In contrast to this, it is much more difficult, especially in older patients, to begin exercise instructions for the first time after they have had surgery. Quadiceps exercises and active assisted range of motion exercises are just as important as training in the use of forearm crutches to allow partial weight bearing on the involved extremity. Partial weight bearing is easily taught by the use of a bathroom scale. In addition to these exercises, general conditioning and especially breathing exercises, are taught.

Operative Technique

A. Supracondylar Osteotomies of the Femur

Supracondylar osteotomy of the femur is the most universal and important corrective osteotomy about the knee. At the same time, however, it is technically the most demanding procedure. This osteotomy allows for correction of varus or valgus deformities, rotational deformities, and specifically, flexion contractures or genu recurvatum. The supracondylar osteotomy is performed at a level in which soft tissues have the largest gliding excursion during joint motion. For this reason, delicate handling of the soft tissues during surgery is especially important. The osteosynthesis has to provide functional stability, and postoperative physical therapy has to begin without delay.

For the stabilization of the supracondylar wedge osteotomy, we have found the AO-blade plates to be the most useful (Fig. 3). In long oblique supracondylar closing wedge osteotomies and in supracondylar opening wedge osteotomies, semitubular plates, specially fashioned at surgery to follow the contour of the bone, provide sufficient stability (Figs. 4 and 5).

Correction of a varus deformity can be accomplished through a lateral approach by the use of a laterally based closing wedge osteotomy internally secured with an AO condylar

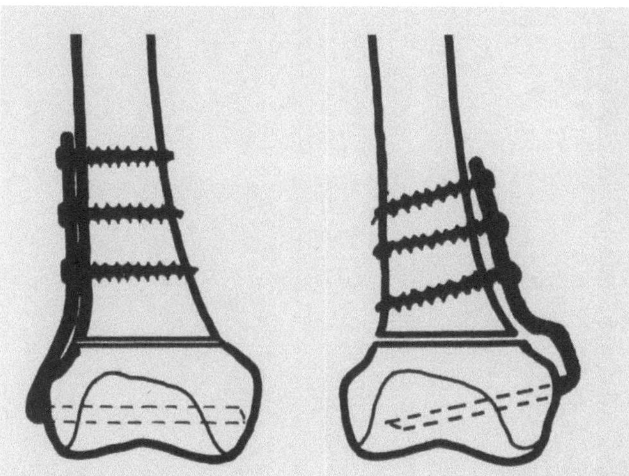

Fig. 3. Schematic drawings demonstrating the principle of osteosynthesis in femoral supracondylar osteotomies. An AO condylar blade plate is used for the lateral approach. An AO 90% blade plate is used from the medial approach. See text for details

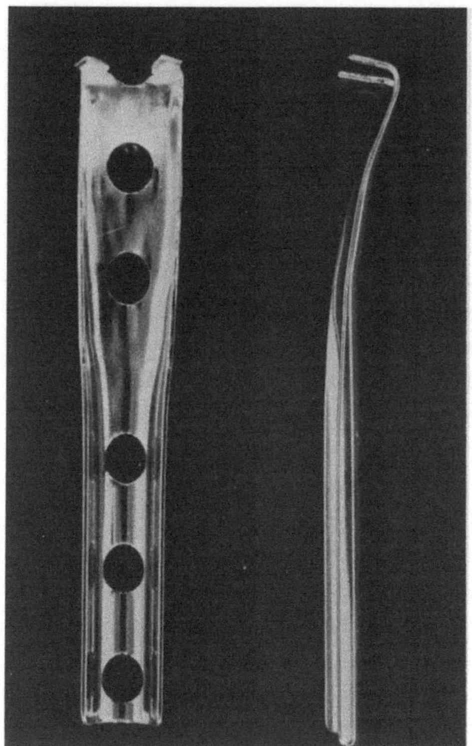

Fig. 4. Photograph of two views of a modified semitubular plate. In difficult osteosynthesis the malleable semitubular plate can be sent to conform with the cortical surface of the bone. Short fragment fixation stability is improved by transformation of the terminal hole into forkshaped hooks for fixation in the cortex

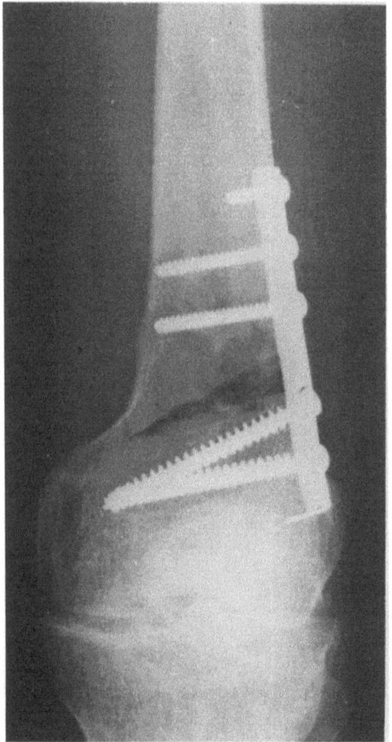

Fig. 5. Radiograph demonstrating a supracondylar opening wedge osteotomy. Axial correction is achieved by opening the osteotomy and bridging it with a seitubular plate. The gaping osteotomy is filled with cancellous bone graft

blade plate. When dealing with osteoporotic bone, the blade frequently has to be inserted more proximally than is normal in fracture treatment. This assures a better fixation of the implant in the metaphyseal cortex. In atrophic bone, the condylar blade plate has the additional advantage that the two most distal screw holes can be filled with cancellous screws which provides significantly better fixation of the device in the distal fragment. In this case, the osteotomy has to be performed at a correspondingly higher level to allow placement of one or two additional screws into the distal fragment depending on the quality of the bone. In supracondylar closing wedge osteotomies in osteoporotic bone, the stability of the osteosynthesis is significantly enhanced by preserving the opposite cortex. Once the plate is fixed to the distal fragment it is then gradually compressed using the AO compression device. By this method, the gaping osteotomy surfaces are approximated while simultaneously achieving axial correction. The intact medial cortex bends gradually to allow for this correction while maintaining its tensile integrity. This serves to protect the medial side of the osteotomy against traction forces. In high metaphyseal osteotomies when the osteotomy plane is horizontal, the medial cortex is relatively thick and fractures under the bending force during closing of the wedge. It is therefore necessary to direct the osteotomy medially and distally aiming for the medial epicondyle so that the medial extent of the osteotomy has its apex against a thinner, more flexible cortex which will deform rather than fracture under the bending stress.

Correction of a valgus deformity is performed through a medial approach using a closing wedge osteotomy and a 90° blade plate (Fig. 3). The same principles which were dis-

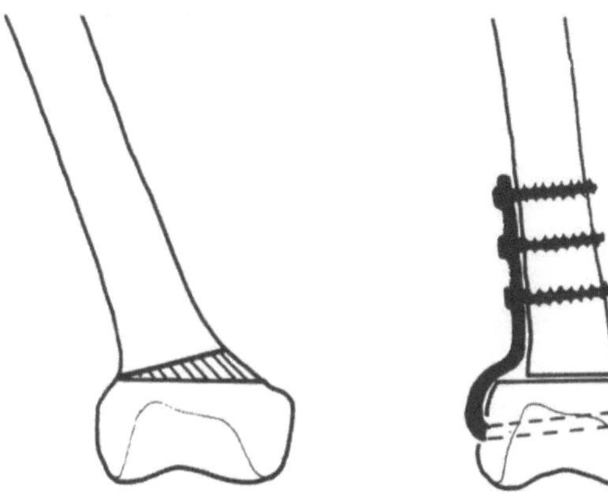

Fig. 6. A and B Schematic drawings demonstrating the supracondylar correction of a severe valgus deformity. The necessary medial displacement of the proximal fragment can be obtained by using a 90° blade plate through a lateral approach. Example **B** demonstrates the failure to achieve satisfactory centralization of the femoral shaft by the use of an AO condylar plate. See text for details

cussed previously for the lateral closing wedge osteotomy, also apply in this situation. The 90° blade plate lends itself especially well to the medial approach because its medial offset conforms well to the distal end of the femur.

The medial approach to the distal femur, however, has three important disadvantages compared to the lateral approach. First, the course of the femoral artery and vein as they exit Hunter's canal make the exposure difficult. Secondly, the skin sensitivity over the medial aspect of the thigh is much greater than laterally and this accounts for the increased pain after the medial approach, and it interferes with physical therapy postoperatively. Finally, in obese patients, the medial approach encounters a much thicker soft tissue layer. For these reasons, it is advantageous to correct a valgus deformity through a lateral approach. The medial approach should be reserved for those exceptional cases where a simultaneous medial arthrotomy is required.

In the correction of a valgus deformity from a lateral approach, the closing wedge osteotomy has to be medially based. It is therefore impossible to leave the medial cortex intact. The 90° blade plate lends itself to osteosynthesis even with a lateral approach because its offset design allows the medial displacement of proximal fragment which is required in the correction of valgus deformities (Fig. 6). Osteosynthesis with a condylar blade plate would align the lateral cortex of the proximal and distal fragments and would shift the axis of the femur over the lateral condyle. The offset design of the 90° blade plate allows for displacement of the proximal fragment medially over the center of the femoral condyles. When dealing with severe valgus deformities, a supracondylar correction may require the use of a 20 mm offset 90° blade plate instead of the standard 10 mm offset plate.

When using 90° blade plates in osteosynthesis, the track for the blade has to be cut into the femoral condyles in a very exacting manner to achieve the intended correction. Because of the relatively large cross section of the blade, any adjustment or redirection after insertion is impossible. During cutting of the blade track the quality of the bone has to be assessed. Dependent upon this quality, one must decide the amount of compression the bone will tolerate and, accordingly, by what amount the blade plate angle will open when tension is applied. This amount of opening must be taken into consideration when cutting the track for the blade.

During alignment of the plate against the proximal femoral fragment, the osteotomy has to have good contact on its opposite cortex while the adjacent cortex gapes and is only brought into contact under increasing compression. When cutting the track for the blade and when performing the osteotomy, care must be taken to avoid fragmentation by first predrilling and then sawing the bone. Forceful seating of the blade edge into the hard cancellous bone of a young patient can cause a fracture of the femoral condyles. Fragmentation of the cortical edge of the osteotomy surface in atrophic bone can compromise stability.

When attempting correction of a valgus deformity through osteoporotic femoral condyles, the stability of the osteosynthesis can be jeopardized when the proximal fragment sinks into the cancellous osteotomy surface of the distal fragment. This danger can be reduced by use of a transverse supracondylar osteotomy at right angles to the femoral shaft instead of a wedge osteotomy. The distal fragment is then placed under the proximal fragment in such a way that the medial corner of the distal fragment is driven into the soft cancellous bone of the proximal fragment. This allows extensive medial cortical contact and provides two point lateral cortical contact to be used in compression with the blade plate (Figs. 5 and 6).

In cases where axial deviation in the frontal plane exists in conjunction with a flexion contracture or a recurvatum deformity, the wedge of the supracondylar osteotomy has to be placed with its base further anteriorly or posteriorly. Accordingly, the blade has to be inserted into the femoral condyles to anticipate this flexion or extension. This allows the plate of the device to be aligned with the femoral shaft after correction has been achieved. In flexion contractures secondary to degenerative arthritis of the knee, an overcorrection to achieve 10° of recurvatum should be attained, otherwise the correction effect will be lost in the first few postoperative days.

The coexistence of an axial deviation with an ipsilateral shortening of the extremity presents an indication for an opening wedge supracondylar femoral osteotomy (Fig. 4). In contrast to the closing wedge osteotomy with excision of a wedge-shaped fragment from the convex side of the deformity, the opening wedge is located on the concave side. The osteotomy is directed toward the opposite epicondyle although the cut is not completed leaving the opposite cortex intact. A semitubular plate is then placed over the open osteotomy site on the concavity of bone and is fixed with screws to the distal fragment. The proximal end of the plate is attached to a distraction apparatus (Distraktion-Spanner by Weller) or laminectomy spreaders are used to gradually open the osteotomy site while the axial deviation is corrected. A lengthening effect of 1–2.5 cm is attained with this technique while a closing wedge osteotomy causes a slight shortening.

The rigidity of the semitubular plate in conjunction with the intact medial cortex provides functional stability. Fixation in the distal fragment can be improved by modification of the plate. The distal hole of a six-hole semitubular plate is cut from the end into a U-shaped fashion with a heavy sheet metal cutter. This gives the end of the plate a U-shape. The two arms of the U are then trimmed along their lateral aspects to make them pointed and give the distal plate a fork-shaped appearance. The two prongs of the fork are bent at right angles toward the concave side of the plate using pliers with smooth jaws (Fig. 5). In performing the osteosynthesis, the two prongs are driven into the bone to provide additional fixation. Two cancellous screws with fully treaded shafts are then placed through the two distal screw holes (Fig. 4).

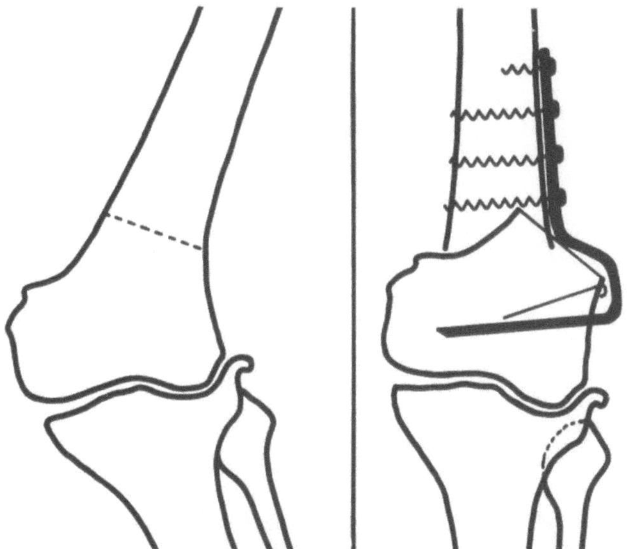

Fig. 7. Schematic drawing illustrating the supracondylar femoral osteotomy for correction of a valgus deformity in advanced osteoporosis. The stability is vastly improved by the medial cortical support offered by this technique.

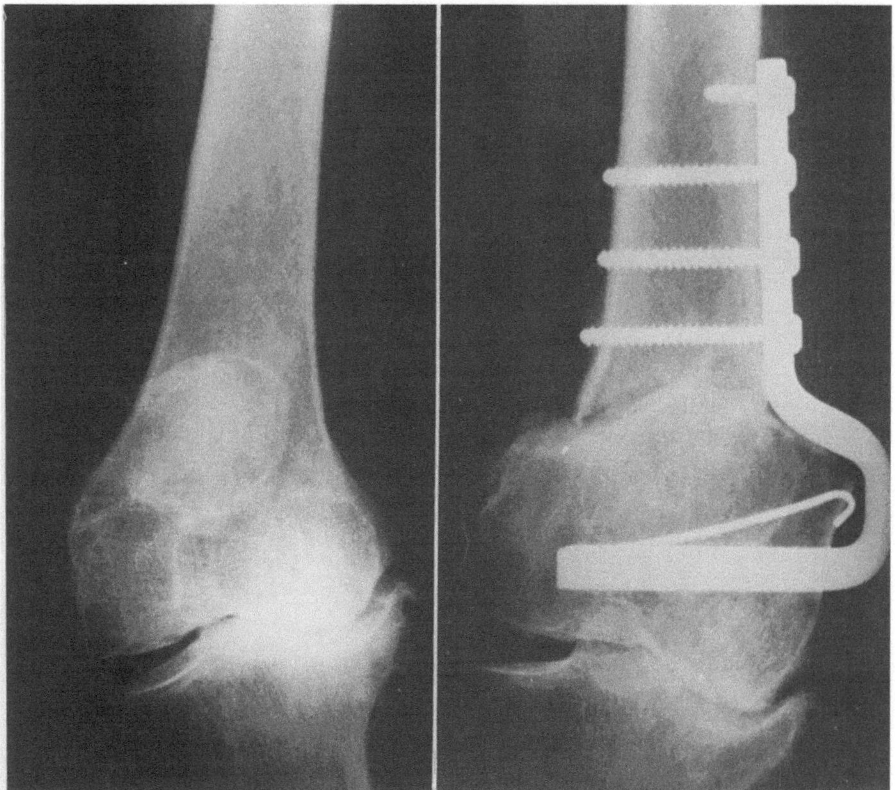

Fig. 8. Radiographs demonstrating the use of the technique described in Figure 7

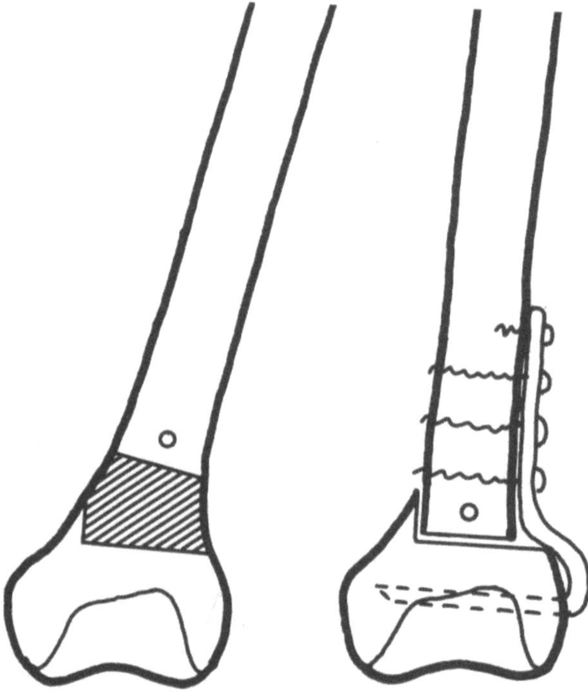

Fig. 9. Schematic drawing illustrating the principle of a femoral supracondylar osteotomy which combines axial correction with shortening. The medial step-cut provides additional stability for the osteosynthesis

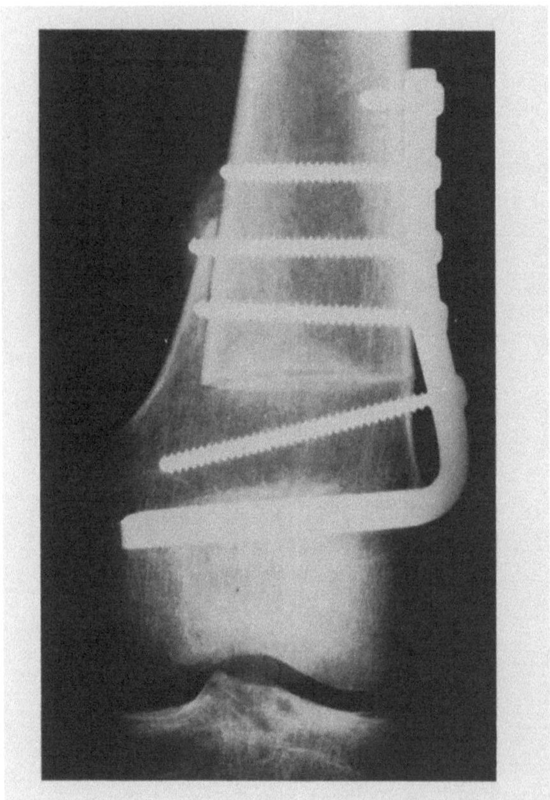

Fig. 10. Radiographs demonstrating the technique described in Figure 9

An accelerated bony consolidation is achieved by covering the gaping osteotomy with a cancellous bone onlay graft. This graft is most conveniently obtained from the cancellous center of the proximal osteotomy surface using a narrow gouge or large currette. The donor site as well as the central portion of the osteotomy gap is packed with Gelfoam before the graft is arranged around the cortex of the osteotomy defect.

In axial malalignment of the distal femur, in an extremity which is longer than the contralateral leg, the supracondylar corrective osteotomy can be combined with a shortening procedure to achieve equalization of leg lengths (Figs. 9 and 10). This can also be utilized in a case where a contralateral fracture has healed with shortening. One has to consider that shortening in the area of the distal femur can result in an insufficient quadiceps mechanism. The shortening should therefore not exceed 3.5 cm. A supracondylar shortening should only be performed when one expects that the patient will be cooperative in the exercise program, and that muscle insufficiency will be eliminated by vigorous training. The relaxation of the musculature resulting from the shortening causes significant loss of stability of the osteosynthesis. Therefore, one should excise the segment of bone in a step-cut fashion leaving the distal medial cortex intact. This acts to provide additional support for the proximal fragment (Fig. 9).

The supracondylar osteotomy also gives an opportunity to correct rotational deformities with relative ease. The distal fragment is simply rotated into its correct alignment prior to performing the osteosynthesis. The degree of rotational correction is limited by the course of the musculature and should not exceed 45°. Rotary realignment in excess of 45° will result in an abnormal direction of muscle action and lead to unphysiological joint function, especially of the patello-femoral joint mechanism.

B. Monocondylar Osteotomies of the Distal Femur and Proximal Tibia

Monocondylar osteotomies are used to correct malunited monocondylar fractures. The procedure is in effect a late reduction. It is performed in conjunction with an arthotomy to allow visualization of the joint surfaces. The knee joint is approached through a medial or lateral parapatellar incision depending on the side of involvement. The incision is extended proximally or distally to allow for application of the osteosynthesis. Starting at the intraarticular step off, the old fracture is carefully reopened. This can usually be accomplished by following the old fracture line. When dealing with small articular fragments, the osteotomy starting at the step off can be directed more vertically toward the diaphysis. This allows the creation of a larger fragment which offers improved conditions for osteosynthesis. In cases of multiple comminuted depressed fragments, the collateral ligaments are incompetent. This incompetence can be corrected by an opening wedge osteotomy in close proximity to the joint surface. If a monocondylar osteotomy is used, the insertion of the collateral ligament is osteotomized with a flake of bone and reinserted under proper tension.

Old fractures invariably show remodeling with rounded edges along the intraarticular step-off covered with a fibrocartilaginous scar. To achieve optimal reduction, the intraarticular edges of the fragments have to be carefully prepared and shaped to allow reconstruction of a smooth, congruent joint surface. The reduced condylar fragment is sta-

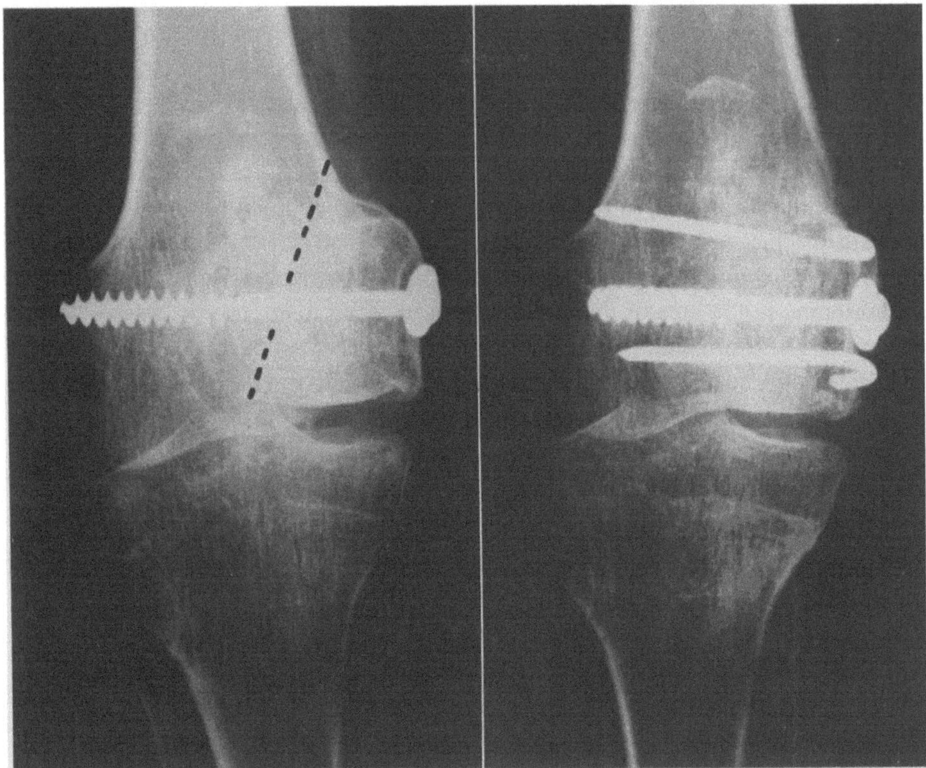

Fig. 11. Radiographs demonstrating an example of a monocondylar femoral osteotomy for correction of malunited intercondylar fractures

bilized by osteosynthesis. A semitubular plate that is fashioned to conform to the surface of the bone provides a good buttress effect. Lag screws placed across the osteotomy site provide interfragmentary compression. When dealing with long osteotomy surfaces, screw fixation by itself might be sufficient. In these cases a minimum of three screws should be used to assure stability in all planes (Figs. 11 and 12).

C. Proximal Tibial Osteotomies

Proximal tibial osteotomy is used to its greatest advantage in varus deformities of the proximal tibia. Obviously, correction of deformity is possible in any plane with a tibial osteotomy, but all others are more difficult and demanding than the correction of a simple varus deformity.

Correction of a valgus deformity requires consideration of the following facts. On the lateral aspect of the leg the investing fascia is placed under increased tension and can lead to a peroneal nerve palsy. In osteotomies to correct valgus deformities, a release of the common peroneal nerve has to be performed concomitantly. The danger is not from traction on the peroneal nerve but rather from direct mechanical pressure on the nerve

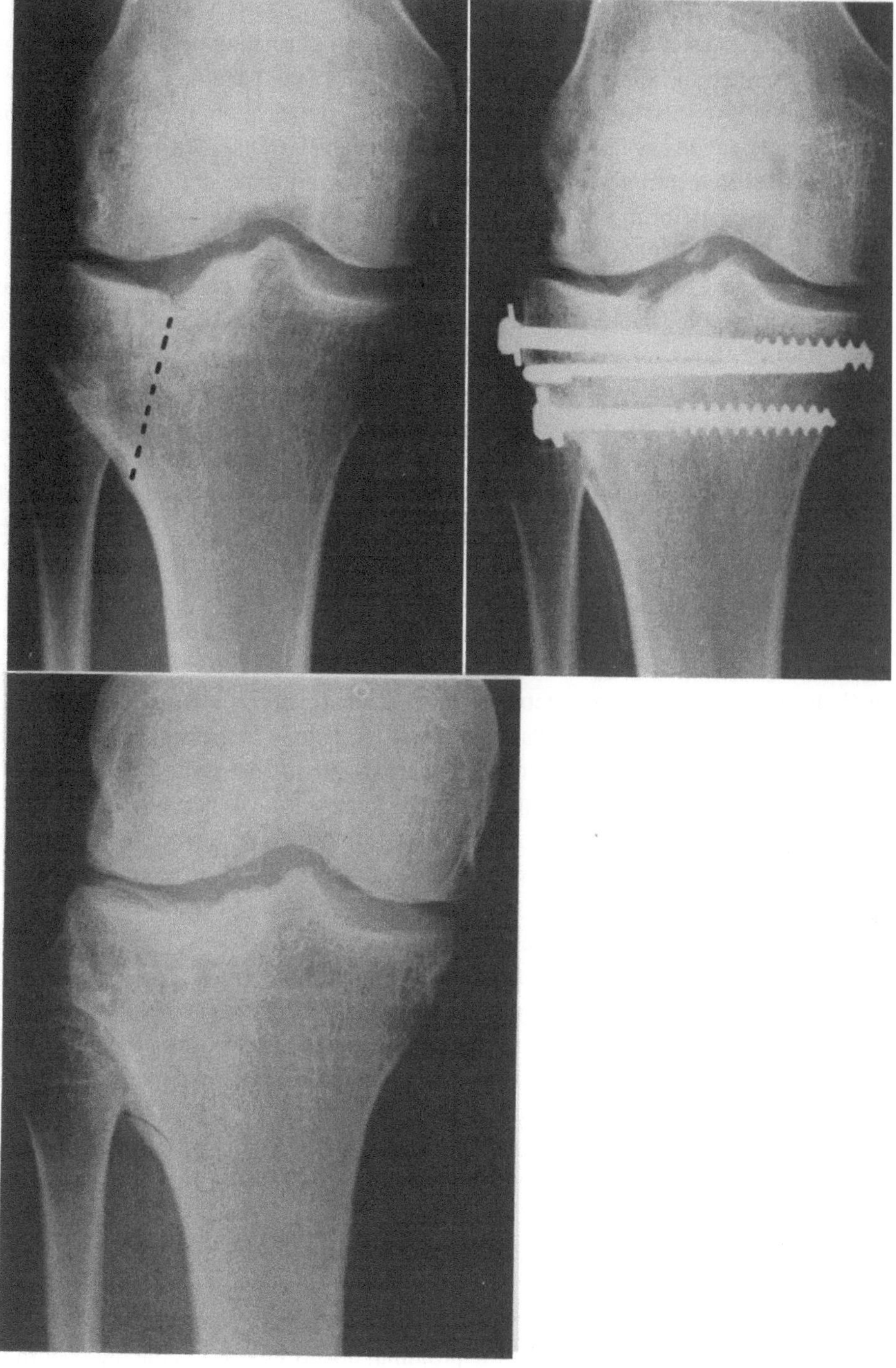

Fig. 12. Radiographs of a twenty year old female. **A** Preoperative radiographs of a malunited lateral tibial plateau fracture 2 years after injury. **B** The same patient eight weeks following monocondylar corrective osteotomy. **C** One year postoperatively

by the tight facia. This leads to compromised vascularity of the nerve and eventually to ischemic nerve damage.

Osteotomies which achieve shortening, correction of rotation or horizontal displacement are limited for anatomic reasons. Skin closure may become a problem after an osteotomy with excessive correction. The anterior compartment musculature requires extensive dissection even for minimal mobilization and is threatened by ischemia, which may progress to a complete anterior compartment syndrome.

A recurvatum deformity is easier to correct than a flexion deformity. This procedure is technically very difficult but allows correction of up to 80°. This can be achieved because the posterior structures are relaxed by the correction while the extensor mechanism can be sufficiently mobilized to allow flexion of the knee. The correction of a significant flexion deformity however produces tension on the posterior structures and threatens damage to the tibial nerve. This procedure has to be performed with great care and only in combination with an adequate shortening of the tibia.

Degenerative arthritis of the knee joint causes a flexion contracture of intraarticular origin but the physiologic posterior tilt of the tibial plateau is maintained. Therefore, the flexion contracture should not be corrected by more than 10° using a proximal tibial osteotomy. Corrections greater than 10° lead to anterior displacement of the femoral condyles on the tibia which results in decreased stability.

All proximal tibial osteotomies require a simultaneous osteotomy of the fibula except minor rotary corrections. The fibula must be osteotomized to decrease its interference with the performance and maintenance of the tibial displacement. It also allows the congruency of the proximal and distal tibiofibular joints to be preserved. The approach is through a longitudinal skin incision over the proximal third of the fibula. The underlying facia is divided in the direction of its fibers. The musculature is bluntly dissected and the fibula is exposed subperiosteally. An oblique osteotomy is performed with careful preservation of the vascular structures on the medial side and the deep peroneal nerve anteriorly.

The following approach for the proximal tibial osteotomy is recommended. A skin incision is made 5 mm lateral and parallel to the anterior tibial crest. The proximal extension curves laterally over the tibial plateau. The fascia is split longitudinally along the tibial crest leaving a narrow rim of fascia for later suturing. The muscles are elevated subperiosteally from the lateral aspect of the tibia. This is accomplished most easily by starting distally to utilize the orientation of the muscle fibers from their origin in the subperiosteal dissection. Of special importance is the dissection of the muscle origin along the flare of the lateral tibial plateau extending close to the fibular head. This avoids traction injury to the muscle at the time of exposure of the lateral aspect of the tibia. Generally this region requires very careful dissection because of its thin soft tissue coverage and the proximity of important neurovascular structures. The use of bulky instruments and implants for osteosynthesis can jeopardize wound healing.

The most advantageous level for the proximal tibia osteotomy is the lower border of the tibial tuberosity. Some of the fibers of the patellar tendon occasionally have to be elevated from their most distal insertions using an osteotome. The high dome or chevron osteotomies proximal to the tibial tubercle create a proximal fragment that is too short to lend itself to stable osteosynthesis. Therefore, these procedures will not be discussed.

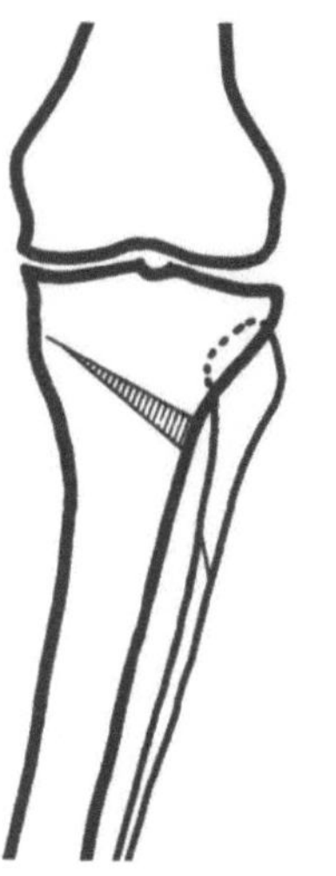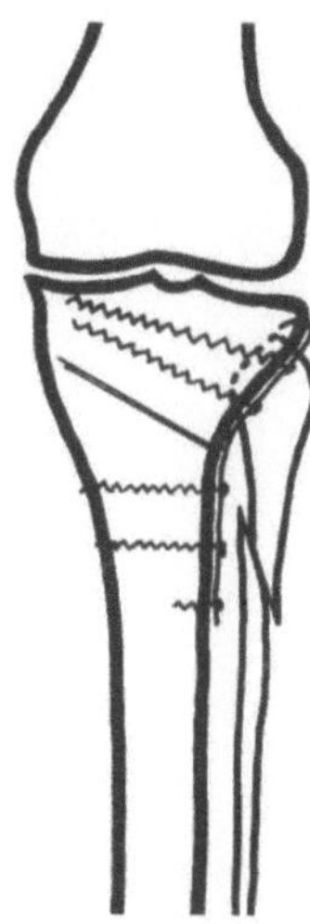

Fig. 13. Drawing demonstrating an oblique closing wedge proximal tibial osteotomy to correct a varus deformity. Note the use of the modified semitubular plate for osteosynthesis

The osteotomy is best performed starting on the lateral aspect of the tibia. A slowly oscillating saw is used and the blade cooled with Ringers solution. The osteotomy must be directed proximally toward a thinner, more flexible cortex on the medial side (Fig. 13). This medial cortex is not transected and is allowed to bend with axial realignment. The preserved cortical continuity over the medial aspect of the tibia resists tensile forces and prevents distraction of the medial side of the osteotomy. The level of this osteotomy corresponds to the pivot point around which the axial deformity has occurred. The base of the wedge to be removed is very narrow due to the small diameter of the bone at this level and because the apex of the wedge does not reach the opposite cortex. A wedge base of 4 mm corresponds to a correction of 10° when done at this level in the tibia. The wedge has to be excised close enough to the opposite apical cortex to allow for bending with closure of the osteotomy and yet not so close that a fracture occurs instead of bending.

A semitubular plate with the fork-shaped modification as described above has proven useful for osteosynthesis of the lateral proximal tibial osteotomy. The proximal portion of the plate is fixed to the tibial plateau fragment utilizing one or two fully threaded cancellous screws. The AO compression device is then attached to the distal end of the plate and while gradual compression is applied the osteotomy gap closes. This results is correction of the axial malalignment. It is important to perform this correction gradually in order to avoid fracture of the intact medial cortex (Fig. 14).

When the proximal tibial osteotomy is used to correct a malrotation, the osteotomy surface is placed horizontally and the opposite cortex has to be fully transected. To stabilize the medial side of the osteotomy, a long cancellous lag screw can be used. This is inserted from the lateral aspect of the distal fragment obliquely into the medial portion of the tibial plateau fragment. It allows compression of the medial portion of the osteotomy (Fig. 15). Compression can be increased by tightening the semitubular plate and the oblique lag screw in an alternating fashion until the desired correction is achieved and the fragments are sufficiently compressed. This same osteosynthesis technique allows

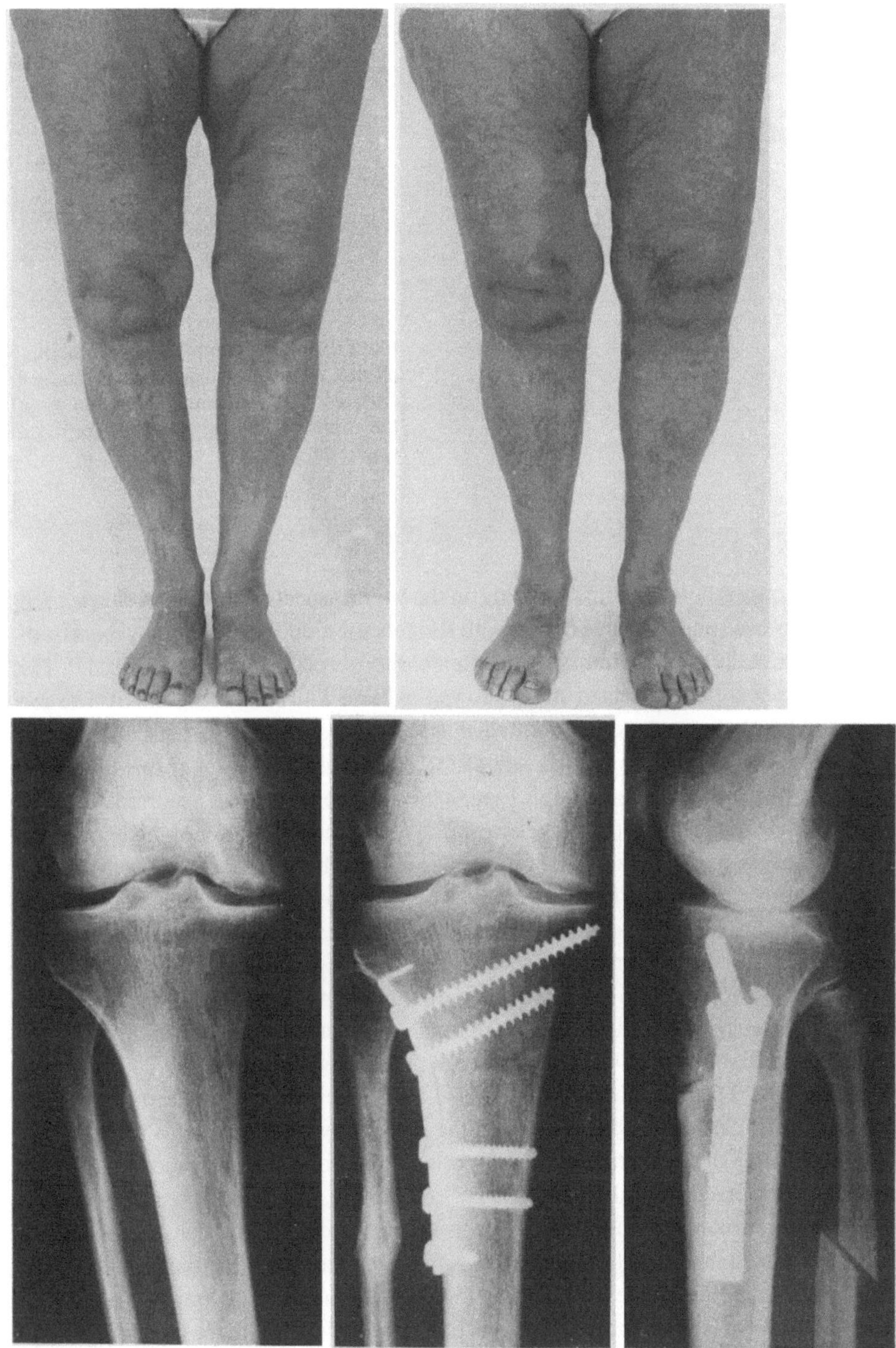

Fig. 14. Clinical example of proximal tibial osteotomy demonstrated in Fig. 13

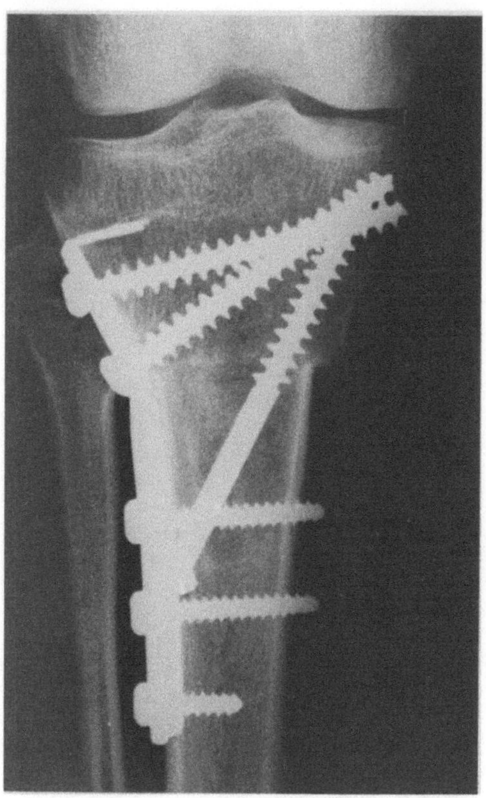

Fig. 15. Radiographs demonstrating a transverse proximal tibial osteotomy for correction of axial and rotational deformity. Osteosynthesis was achieved with the specially modified semitubular plate. Medial stabilization was obtained using the oblique cancellous lag screw

correction of a valgus deformity through a lateral approach to the proximal tibia. The difference between this technique and that for correction of a varus deformity is that the wedge must be based medially. To correct additional flexion or recurvatum deformities, the base of the osteotomy wedge has to be placed further anteriorly or posteriorly.

The wound closure requires that great care must be taken not to close the muscle fascia under tension in order to prevent an anterior compartment syndrome. If necessary, the fascia must be incised in a relaxing fashion at multiple levels and sometimes closure of the fascia has to be deleted entirely.

Finally, correction of a valgus deformity can be achieved by a medial approach through a longitudinal skin incision along the medial tibial crest. Osteosynthesis requires the same considerations as it does for the lateral osteotomy. Correction of a valgus deformity through either approach carries the danger of peroneal nerve damage thus making a relaxing incision of the fascia overlying the nerve mandatory in either case. Osteotomies from the medial approach require relaxation of the anterior fascia of the leg to safeguard against a compartment syndrome (Fig. 16).

D. Corrective Osteotomies of the Tibial Shaft

Axial malalignment in the diaphyseal area occurs mostly as a result of malunited fractures. The deleterious biomechanical effect of such deformities is not diminished by their distance from the knee. Axial malalignment of the tibial shaft can only be corrected

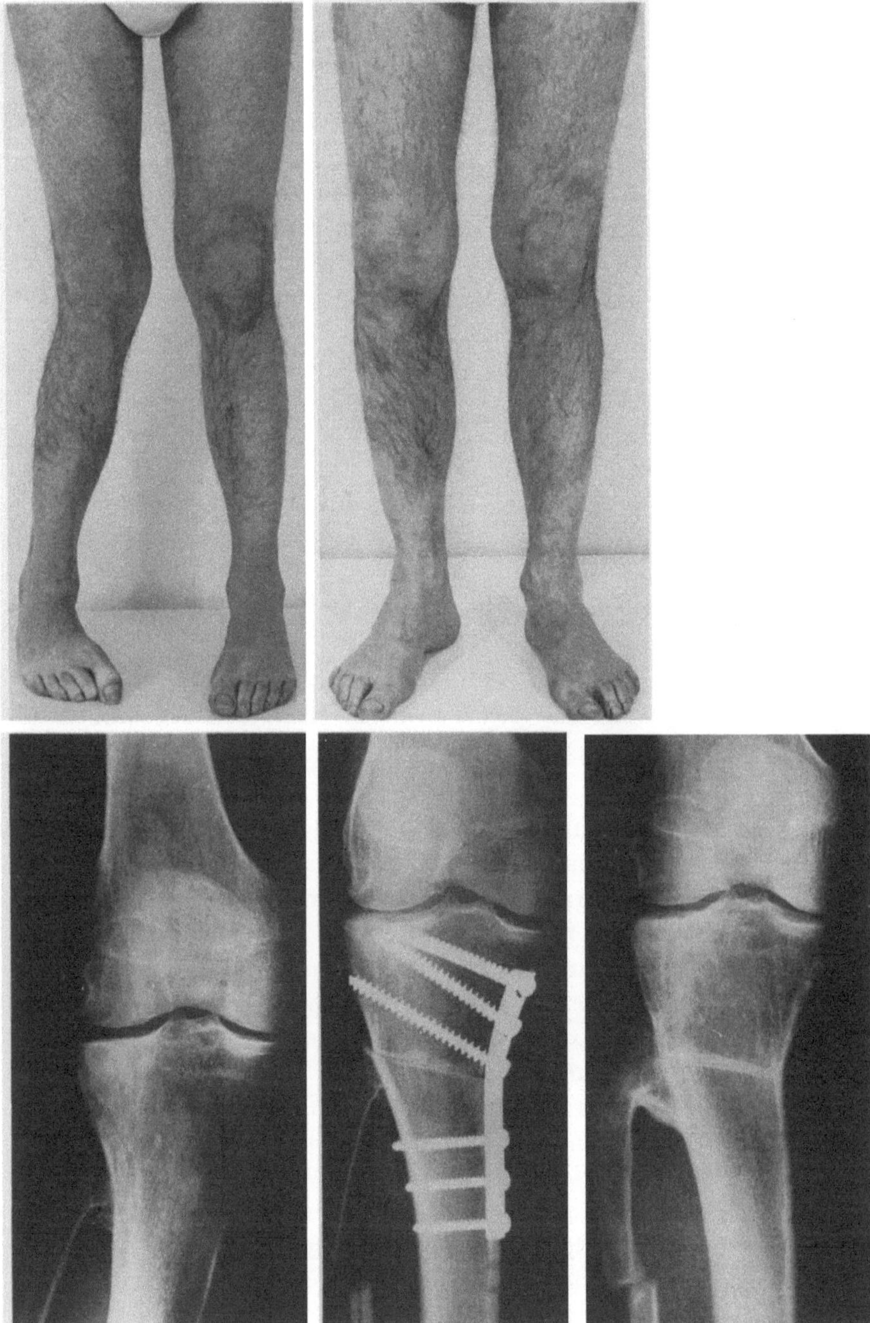

Fig. 16. Clinical example of an upper tibial osteotomy for correcting valgus deformity. A medial bone wedge has been removed and the osteotomy has been stabilized by using a semitubular plate. Additionally the peroneal nerve has been released (male age 51 years, before and 2 years after surgery

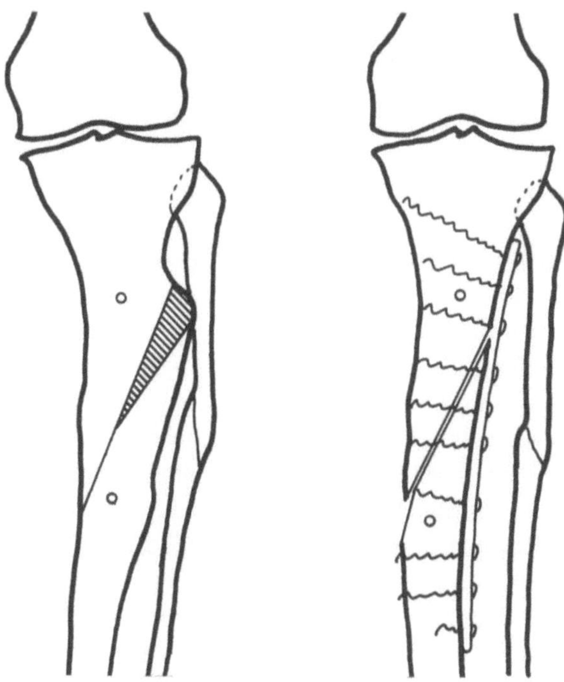

Fig. 17. Schematic drawing illustrating the principle of a long oblique osteotomy through the tibial diaphysis. This technique allows some lenthening together with axial correction. Osteosynthesis is obtained with lag screws and a neutralization plate

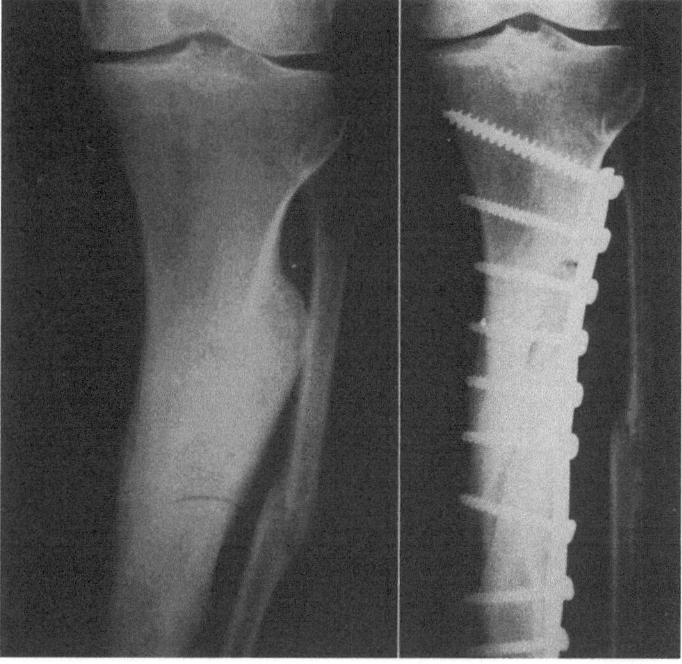

Fig. 18. Radiographs demonstrating the technique illustrated in Figure 17

to a limited degree through metaphyseal osteotomies. Corrections close to the knee offer the advantage that they are performed through cancellous bone and, therefore, have better conditions for bony healing. Their disadvantage lies in the fact that they create an additional compensatory curve resulting in an S-shaped bone. Also, they do not offer correction of the abnormal biomechanical effects on the ankle joint. Special local conditions in the area of deformity such as severe scarring, extensive soft tissue loss, or chronic osteomyelitis in the area of the malunion, may prohibit surgery in this region. A metaphyseal osteotomy may be, therefore, the only available choice for correction of the malalignment. However, if tissue conditions at the malunion site permit, a diaphyseal osteotomy at this level should be performed. This restores the normal anatomical relationships and is biomechanically the best solution.

The technique of the diaphyseal osteotomy must take into account the shape of the bone at the apex of the deformity as well as the type of malalignment. One must evaluate the need to correct rotation or shortening while realigning the axial deformity. All variations of diaphyseal osteotomies have to be planned in consideration of the special conditions that exist in the healing of cortical bone and of the surrounding soft tissues.

The diaphyseal wedge osteotomy requires exposure of the bone at the osteotomy site by decortication. At the apex of the deformity a wedge with its base toward the convexity is excised. While correcting the deformity, the gaping osteotomy site is closed and stabilized using AO compression plating over the former convexity. In performing the osteosynthesis, it is important to assure that the osteotomy gap remains closed on the side

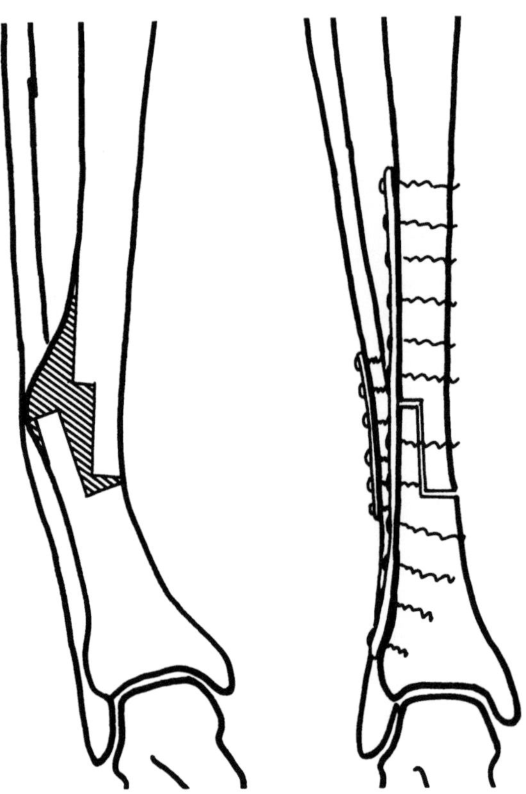

Fig. 19. Schematic drawing to illustrate Figure 20 showing a step-cut diaphyseal osteotomy of the tibia for axial correction. Osteosynthesis is obtained with lag screws and a compression plate

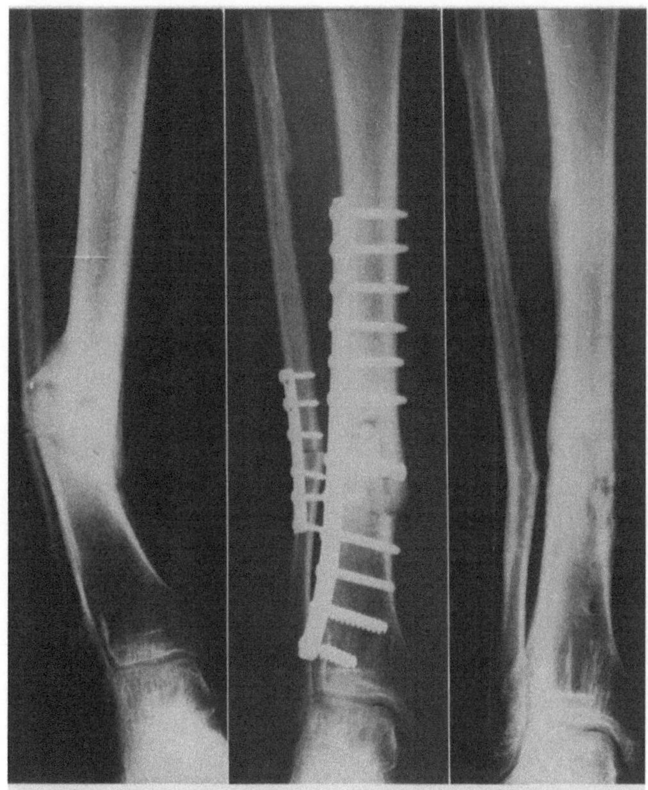

Fig. 20. A step-cut diaphyseal osteotomy of the tibia for axial correction. (Male 35 years of age, final radiogram 2 years after osteotomy)

opposite the plate. This is done to assure compression and avoid fatigue fracture of the plate. If this can not be achieved, the plate must be bent at the level of the osteotomy site in the direction of the old deformity. This will then provide close contact of the osteotomy fragments. All transverse osteotomies through the diaphysis should have autologous cancellous bone grafts placed across the osteotomy site. Without grafting, consolidation may be delayed.

If diaphyseal wedge osteotomies are used to correct rotational deformities at the same time, this becomes technically easier when one of the osteotomy planes is placed perpendicular to the shaft. This will assure that rotational correction will not be translated into axial deviation.

A malunion which shows a prominent bulbous deformity is best corrected by utilizing a long oblique wedge osteotomy. This allows a larger surface area of bony contact between the fragments and greater interfragmentary pressure can be applied by the use of lag screws. The stabilization of an oblique osteotomy is achieved through the use of lag screws with a neutralization plate. The lag screws may be placed through screw holes in the plate or outside the plate (Figs. 17 and 18). When dealing with abundant bone stock one can use a step-cut corrective osteotomy. In this case a compression plate should be used in addition to lag screws (Figs. 19 and 20).

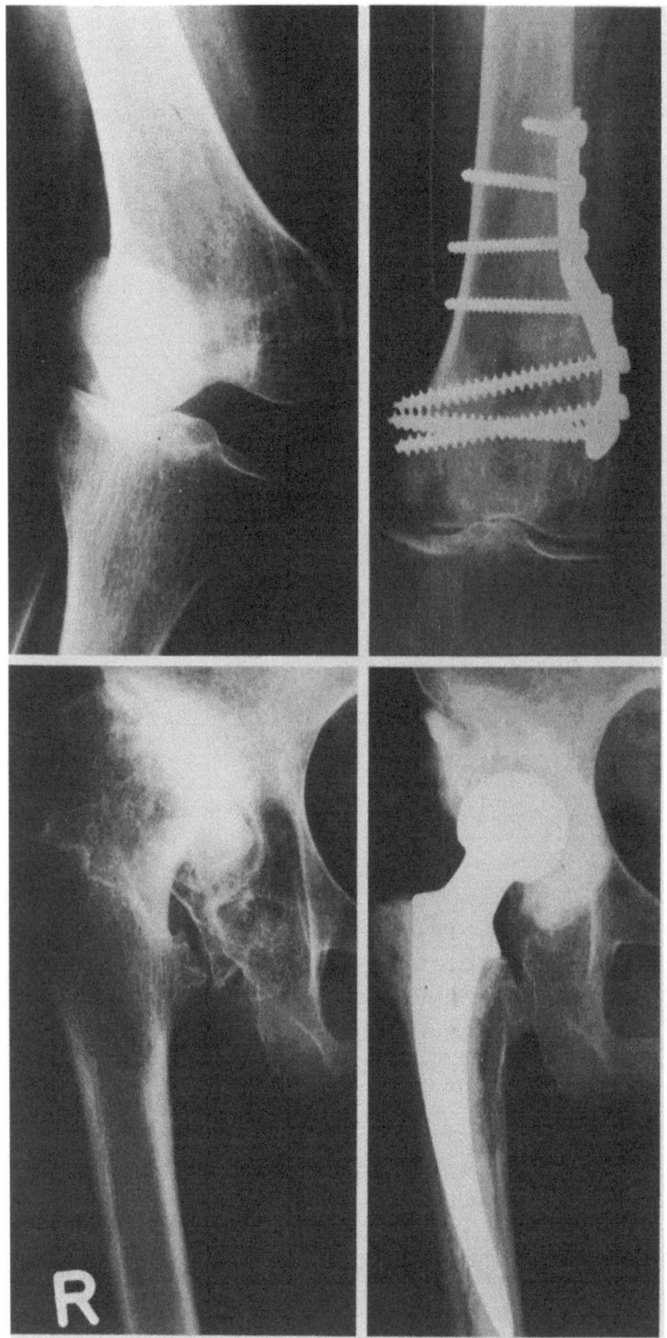

Fig. 21. Osteoarthrosis and valgus-instability of the knee joint caused by an adduction-contracture of the ipsilateral osteoarthritic hip. The correction of the deformity required supracondylar osteotomy, revision of the knee joint with ligament repair and total hip replacement (female at age 56, before and 5 years after surgery)

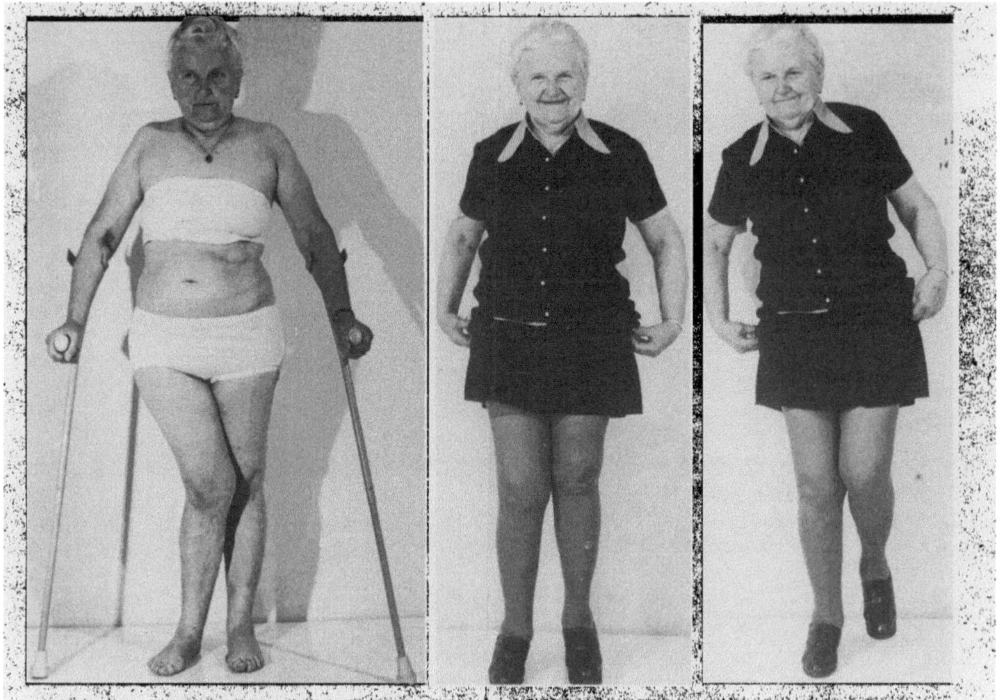

Fig. 22. The same case as demonstrated in Fig. 21, before and 5 years after surgery

E. Correction of Hip Malalignment in Osteoarthrosis of the Knee

Degenerative osteoarthritis of the knee joint not only occurs as a result of malalignment about the knee but may also develop as sequellae of a tight hip joint in poor position. A partial or complete fusion of the hip joint in excessive abduction or adduction leads to medial or lateral stresses on the knee. In time, this stress may cause arthrotic changes with progressive varus or valgus deformities even in a knee that was previously normal. In this situation, an attempt to influence the progressive arthrotic malalignment by a corrective osteotomy about the knee is futile while the abnormal stresses on the knee persist. Correction of the malpositioned hip or improvement of hip mobility by appropriate means are mandatory before this variant of osteoarthritis of the knee can be successfully treated by corrective osteotomy (Figs. 21 and 22).

Summary

The indications and techniques of the most important corrective osteotomies for treatment of degenerative osteoarthritis of the knee are described. Stable osteosynthesis allows accurate correction and immediate postoperative physical therapy. This enabled the corrective osteotomies to gain great clinical importance. These procedures are technically demanding but, if successfully performed, will delay progression of arthrotic changes and improve the functional stability of the malaligned knee joint. This assures satisfying, long-lasting results. The beneficial effects of these osteotomies should not be disregarded and they will frequently negate the need for total knee replacement and will invariably postpone prosthetic replacement.

Acknowledgement: The author gratefully acknowledges Roger W. Hood, M.D., Boston, Mass., and Winfried M. Berger, M.D., LTC MC USA, Altdorf bei Nürnberg, West Germany, for translating this paper.

References

Allgöwer M, Kinzl L, Matter P, Perren SM, Rüedi T (1973) Die dynamische Kompressionsplatte. Springer, Berlin Heidelberg New York

Fischer S (1972) Operative Beinverkürzung und Beinverlängerung. Orthopäde 1:50

Hafner E, Meuli HCh (1975) Röntgenuntersuchung in der Orthopädie. Huber, Bern Stuttgart Wien

Heidensohn P, Hohmann D, Weigert M (1972) Subtrochantere Verkürzungs- und Verlängerungs-osteotomie. Orthopäde 1:46

Heim U, Pfeiffer KM (1972) Periphere Osteosynthesen. Springer, Berlin Heidelberg New York

Müller ME (1971) Die hüftnahen Femurosteotomien. II. Aufl. Thieme, Stuttgart

Müller ME, Allgöwer M, Willenegger H (1969) Manual der Osteosynthese, Springer, Berlin Heidelberg New York

Pflüger W (1972) Erfahrungen mit der operativen Unterschenkelverlängerung nach Anderson. Orthopäde 1:57

Wagner H (1972) Technik und Indikation der operativen Verkürzung und Verlängerung von Ober- und Unterschenkel. Orthopäde 1:59

Translated from the German: Wagner H (1977) Korrekturosteotomien am Bein. Orthopäde 6:145–177 © Springer Verlag 1977

Gait Analysis and its Benefit to the Patient

J.U. Baumann

Indication for and evaluation of treatment in diseases and traumatic conditions of the locomotor system logically should include assessment of the quality of locomotor function. The orthopaedic surgeon relies on the case history, radiological evaluation, and on testing movements on the examining table. He usually observes the gait pattern while the patient enters and leaves the examination room. Such a procedure is often inadequate for assessing a function which depends on complicated interactions of neural commands and transmissions, muscle contractions and simultaneous angular changes in many joints. As a rule, the locomotor function is affected as a whole even when there is only a minor localised lesion.

Gait inspection is presumed to provide all necessary informations. However there are several reasons why this is unsatisfactory, if additional pertinent information is not obtained.

In order to properly observe locomotor patterns, the patient should be viewed from the front, back and side. To permit this, an examination area measuring at least 6 × 6 meters is required. In daily orthopaedic practice, this can rarely be fulfilled.

Important gait sequences occur too fast to be seen in detail. This applies particularly to the period of bilateral foot support and when observing the patient from the side.

Concomitant angular joint changes cannot be observed simultaneously or compared with each other, except as a general impression of harmony of movement.

Gait inspection only allows evaluation of positional changes of body segments. It is impossible to perceive underlying internal and external forces.

Diseases and traumatic conditions of the locomotor system represent one of the most important causes of long term working disability in the United States (White 1973). Therefore there is no doubt, that objective measurements, in addition to simple clinical judgement of the quality of gait, are desirable.

Since the 16th century attempts have been made to overcome the physical limitations in observing and describing gait patterns, but they have only become successful since the invention of photography. These investigations were even an important incentive for the development of cinematography (Marey 1873). Progress in electronic technology renders it possible to apply the pioneer work done in Europe by Braune and Fischer (1895-1904) and by Scherb (1952), by Elftman (1939), Eberhart and Inman (1954) and Schwartz and Heath (1964) in North America – to name some investigators – on a day to day basis.

The factor of cost-efficiency of modern gait analysis must be considered in regard to the phenomenon of cost explosion in medicine.

The increase of biomechanical knowledge of the locomotor system and the general application of available information should have a long term effect on the efficacy of the expensive therapy required today by a high percentage of the overaging population in Europe and North America:

Endoprosthetic joint replacement is burdened by the problems of long term fixation requiring a large number of expensive reoperations.

More detailed knowledge concerning the physiology and pathophysiology of weight bearing on human joints would probably help to reduce the number of such failures (Crowninshield et al. 1978; Murray et al. 1972).

Rotational joint movements around vertical axes are probably essential for the economy of human gait and may represent a major factor in endoprosthetic loosening. Their amplitude and speed in different age groups of patients with normal and pathologic joints is only poorly understood.

Proper indications for therapeutic exercises, orthoses and surgical interventions for patients suffering from cerebral palsy, myelodysplasia and neuromuscular diseases are only partially known. Long term follow-up controls based on reliable documents including gait analysis are beginning to shed some light on this problem (Baumann et al. 1978; Perry 1974; Simon et al. 1978; Sutherland and Cooper 1978).

Similar situations exist in other orthopaedic fields (De Weerd et al. 1977).

The possibilities and laws of physiologic compensations for localised disturbances of movements or of joint loading are only guessed at today. In spite of their practical significance they are largely unknown (Johnson and Waugh 1979).

Energy expenditure for locomotion is a good indicator for the efficiency of the locomotor system. So far, its measurement as a basis for evaluation of a patient's condition and treatment is infrequently applied in daily practice but it would be desirable (Arborelius et al. 1976).

Useful instruments are available to solve these problems (Fig. 1). Progress in electronics promises improvement in accuracy and simplicity. The initial cost of the instruments is still high but it should be possible to keep operating expenses relatively low. The expense for examinations must not exceed those of customary radiological examinations. Concentration on the solution of actual problems of the individual with proper selection of the procedure by gait analysis may be a key factor in keeping expenses down. This judgement can only be made by a clinician.

Today the following techniques are used in gait analysis:

1. Spatial measurement of the position of body segments and of joint angles between them at regular time intervals by:
- Cinephotography,
- Chronocyclophotography with reflecting or self-illuminated measuring targets (Selspot-System, TV-Computer-Interface),
- Goniometry (Electro-Goniometry, Polarized-Light-Goniometry).
2. Dynamometry of external forces:
- Measuring ground reaction forces by force-plates or mats. A variety of different me-

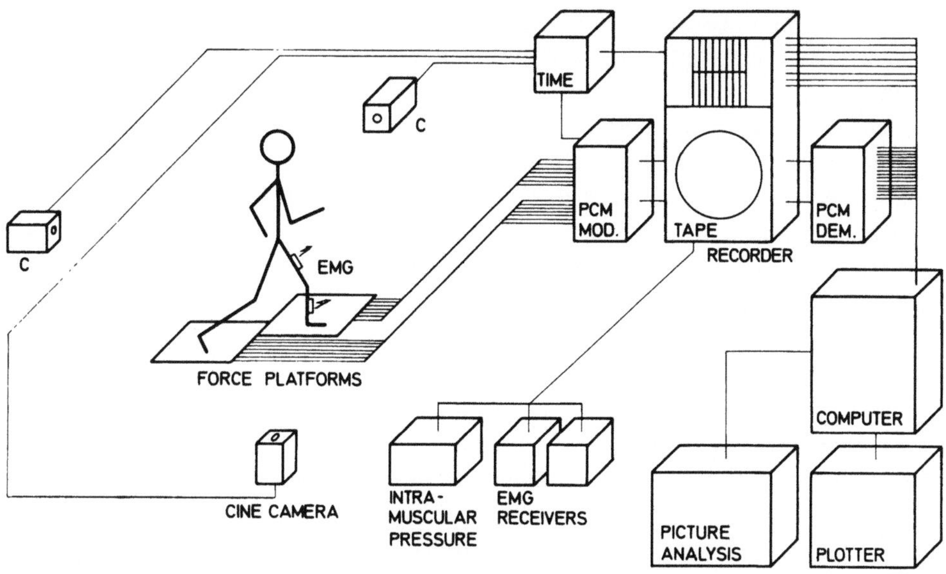

Fig. 1. Instrumentation for gait analysis including cinephotography, telemetered electromyography, and force plates. It is not always necessary to use the entire system to solve particular clinical questions. (EMG = Electromyography, PCM = Pulse code modulation, MOD = Modulator, DEM = Demodulator)

chano-electrical transducers are available, piezo-electric systems are most frequently used,
– Force transducers built into shoes,
– Accelerometry.
   3. Dynamometry of internal forces:
– Evaluation of active and passive muscle forces and tensions, by electromyography and measurement of intramuscular pressure as an indicator of tension (Baumann et al. 1979).
– Evaluation of joint forces and loads by calculation from correlated force-plate and kinematic data.
– Direct measurement of joint forces and loads by telemeterized endoprostheses.
   4. Ergometry:
– Measurement with Douglas bag, gas analysis,
– Calculation from force-plate data (Cavagna 1975).

In most instances gait analysis is a non-intrusive method without any potentially harmful irradiation. To provide useful results, the methods must not impair the patient's freedom of movement.

The results must be presented in a form which is easily understood by the average clinician. Results usually include the following information which should be available within a few hours after testing:

1. Walking speed, step length, duration of stance and swing phase for each leg.
2. Angular degree values for hip, knee and ankle joints, pelvic obliquity, pelvic tilt and pelvic rotation as well as their progression during one or several gait cycles.

3. Foot-to-floor reaction forces in the sagittal, frontal, and horizontal planes with the point of impact of the vertical force on the foot sole and the moment of transverse foot rotation.
– Changing values of these forces during repetitive measurements.
– The moments produced by external forces on hip, knee, and ankle joint as calculated from force vectors and their spatial relationship to joint axes.

4. Intensity and activity periods of individual muscles which are important under specific conditions as discerned by electromyography. Activity periods must be compared with related joint movements and foot-to-floor forces.

5. Total energy requirement for locomotion.
– Changing levels of potential energy, translational kinetic energy and rotational kinetic energy concerning individual body segments.

For more than 12 years the use of gait analysis by cinephotography with 50 exposures per second and exposure times of 2–6 milliseconds has provided the author with a basis for indications or contraindications for physiotherapeutic measures, orthotes and operations in patients with cerebral palsy. Profound changes in outlining a treatment plan have been the result. Similar progress can be expected for other fields of orthopaedics in the future, particularly for patients suffering from arthrosis of hip and knee joints. Knowledge concerning the influence of different body proportions on joint configuration during dynamic loading may lead to more successful operations for biomechanical realignement as well as for prevention of joint impairment due to excessive wear.

Acknowledgement: Work supported by Swiss National Research Fund Credit No. 3.984.78

References

Arborelius MM, Carlsson AS, Nilsson BE (1976) Oxygen Intake and Walking Speed before and after Total Hip Replacement. Clin Orthop 121:113

Baumann JU, Meyer E, Schürmann K (1978) Hip Adductor Transfer to the Ischial Tuberosity in Spastic and Paralytic Hip Disorders. Arch Orthop Traumat Surg 92:107

Baumann JU, Sutherland DH, Hänggi A (1979 in print) Intramuscular Pressure during Walking. An Experimental Study using the Wick Catheter Technique. Clin Orthop

Braune CW, Fischer O (1895–1904) Der Gang des Menschen. Abh. d. math.-phys. Kl. d. königl. Sächs. Ges. d. Wiss. Vol. 21, 25, 26, 28, Leipzig

Cavagna GA (1975) Force Platforms as Ergometers. J Appl Physiol 39:174

Crowninshield RD, Johnston RC, Andrews JB, Brant RA (1978) A Biomechanical Investigation of the Human Hip. J Biomech Vol II:75

De Weerd JH (Jr.), Stauffer RN, Chao EY, Axmear FE (1977) Functional Evaluation of pre- and postoperative Total Knee Arthoplasty Patients. Orthop Trans 1:54

Eberhart HD, Inman VT, Bresler BP (1954) The Principal Elements in Human Locomotion. In: Human Limbs and Their Substitutes, p. 437 Ed. Klopsteg + Wilson, McGraw-Hill Book Co., New York

Elftman H (1939) Forces and Energy Changes in the Leg during Walking. Amer J Physiol 125, 339

Johnson F, Waugh W (1979) Method for Routine Clinical Assessment of Knee Joint Forces. Med Biol Eng Combut 17:145

Marey EJ (1873) La Machine Animale. Locomotion Terrestre (bipedes). Ballière, Paris

Murray MP, Brewer BJ, Zuege RC (1972) Kinesiologic Measurement of Functional Performance Before and After McKee-Farrar Total Hip Replacement. J Bone Joint Surg 54-A:237
Perry J (1974) Kinesiology of Lower Extremity Bracing. Clin Orthop 102:18
Simon SR, Deutsch SD, Nuzzo RM, Mansour MJ, Jackson JL, Koskinen M, Rosenthal RK (1978) Genu Recurvatum in Spastic Cerebral Palsy. Report on Findings by Gait Analysis. J Bone Joint Surg 60-A:882
Sutherland DH, Cooper L (1978) The Pathomechanics of Progressive Crouch Gait in Spastic Diplegia. Orthop Clin of North America 9:143
Scherb R (1952) Kinetisch-diagnostische Analyse von Gehstörungen. Enke, Stuttgart
Schwartz RP, Heath AL, Morgan DW, Towns RC (1964) A Quantitative Analysis of Recorded Variables in the Walking pattern of "Normal" Adults. J Bone Joint Surg 46-A:324
White KL (1973) Life and Death in Medicine. Sc Am 229:23

Conservative Orthopaedic Management of Children with Myelomeningoceles

K. Schürmann, J.U. Baumann

Today patients with congenital anomalies of the spine and spinal cord in the form of myelomeningoceles often live to middle age or even longer. They suffer from flaccid parapareses, which are often combined with spastic components. These children can usually be taught to walk with orthoses and other orthopaedic devices. Without these aids, ambulation is often impossible or at least strenuous. Orthoses are orthopaedic appliances that act as an external skeleton. They permit axial loading of the trunk and lower limbs by replacing missing muscular stabilisation. By achieving the ability to stand and walk, complications resulting from being bedridden or from continuous sitting in a wheel chair, e.g. decubiti, demineralization, osteoporosis as well as pathological fractures, can be avoided.

Material

All 41 patients with myelomeningoceles of age 3 or more who are at present being treated in the Neuro-Orthopaedic Unit of the Children's Hospital of Basel have been examined with emphasis on the use of orthoses. The age distribution is given in Table 1. At the time

Table 1. Age distribution

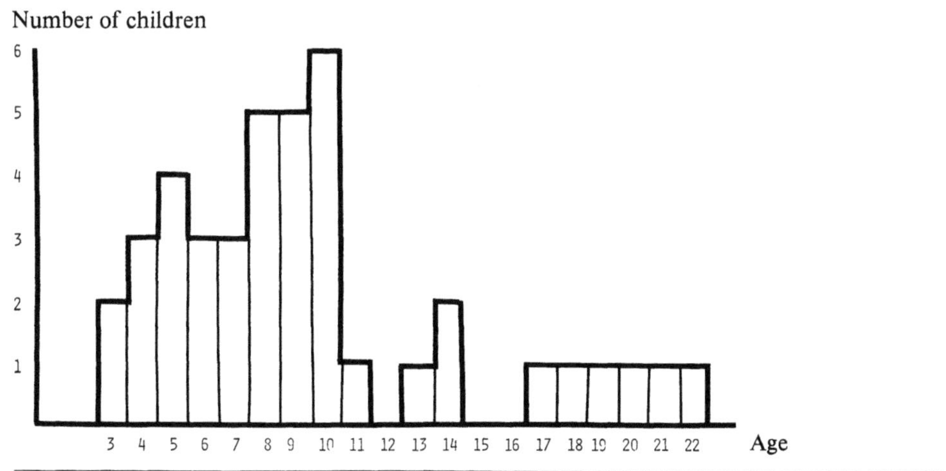

Table 2. Upper level of lesion

Th 12	1 child
L1/L2	9 children
L3/L4	16 children
L5	11 children
sacral	4 children

of investigation the youngest was 3 and the oldest 22 years old. There were 20 boys and 21 girls. The level of the lesion is given in Table 2. The patients were grouped according to their functional ability by the classification of Hoffer et al. (1973).

Orthoses

The following types of orthoses were used:
1. ankle-foot-orthoses
2. knee-ankle-foot-orthoses
3. hip-knee-ankle-foot-orthoses ("myelomeningocele-orthoses")

Ankle-foot-orthoses were used for lesions involving the lower lumbar and sacral spinal cord. In these patients, the musculature responsible for the movement of hip and knee joints is sufficiently strong. The main problem is instability as a result of paralysis of the muscles of the lower leg and foot. Calcaneus deformities were prevalent. They were combined with either varus or valgus deformities. Therefore solid ankle orthoses of polypropylene were prescribed most frequently (Fig. 1a, b). These orthoses are light in weight

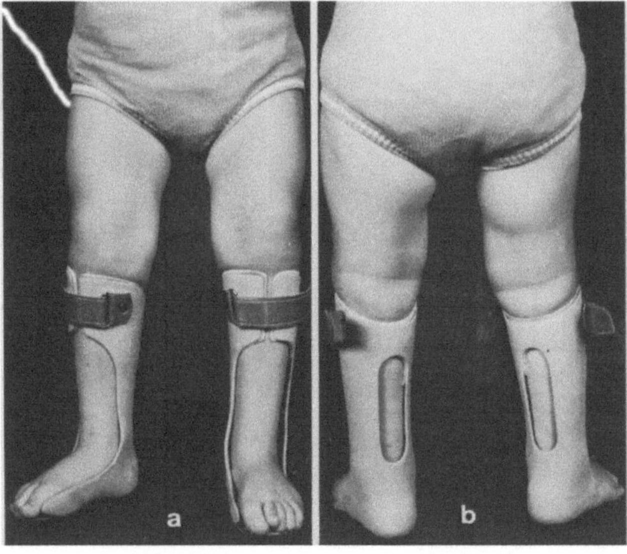

Fig. 1a and b. Ankle-foot orthosis of polypropylene with solid ankle. Normal shoes can be worn

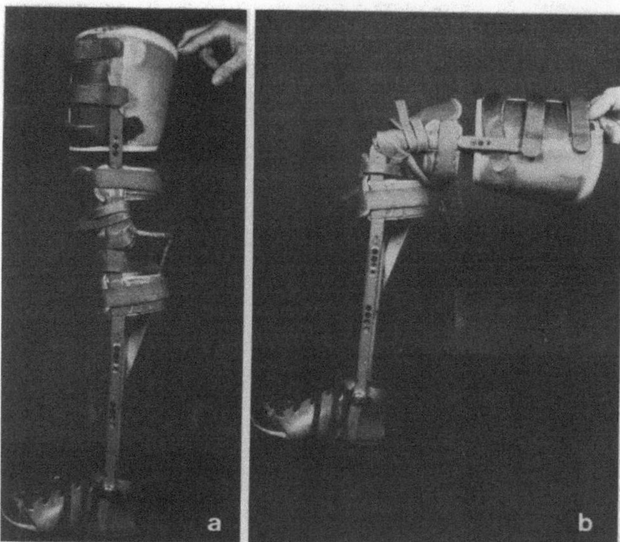

Fig. 2a and b. Conventional double-bar above knee orthosis (knee-ankle-foot orthosis) with knee lock, ankle joints, metal and leather shoe insert for use in paralysis of the foot and knee when the hip musculature is sufficiently strong

and can be used with various shoe types including gym shoes. So-called "inner shoes" of leather strengthened with plastic material are in use in some parts of Europe for the above mentioned deformities. These "inner shoes" are preferred in some centers because of the non skin irritating properties of the leather. The polypropylene orthosis of Lindseth and Glancy (1974) has the advantage of not completely enclosing the leg, resulting in less restriction of blood circulation and reduction of hyperthermia.

Both types of orthoses stabilize the talo-crural and subtalar joints. The shoes used in conjunction with them should have rounded or cushioned heels as well as a rocker sole to compensate for the lack of function of the talo-crural joint. Patients who have to walk up and down inclines prefer a conventional double bar ankle-foot-orthosis with stops for dorsi- and plantar flexion. Knee-ankle-foot-orthoses are required for patients with insufficient stability of the knee while standing or walking. As a rule, these patients have neurologic lesions at the level of L4/L5. In these cases the knee musculature is partially functional.

Two types of long leg braces should be considered: a long leg double bar orthosis with knee lock is given to young children (Fig. 2a, b). Later it is often possible to prescribe a mobile knee joint with assisted extension in the form of rubber bands in place of the knee lock. This allows restricted knee flexion during the swing phase and results in a more natural gait which probably reduces the energy output necessary for forward motion.

For these knee-ankle-foot-orthoses there are 3 possibilities to stabilize the foot:
1. The use of a caliper attached to specially adapted shoes.
2. The use of ankle joints with stops for dorsi- and plantar flexion and a shoe insert.
3. A molded plastic solid ankle shell for lower leg and foot. The shoes worn with the orthosis must compensate for the stiff ankle joint with cushion heels and rocker soles.

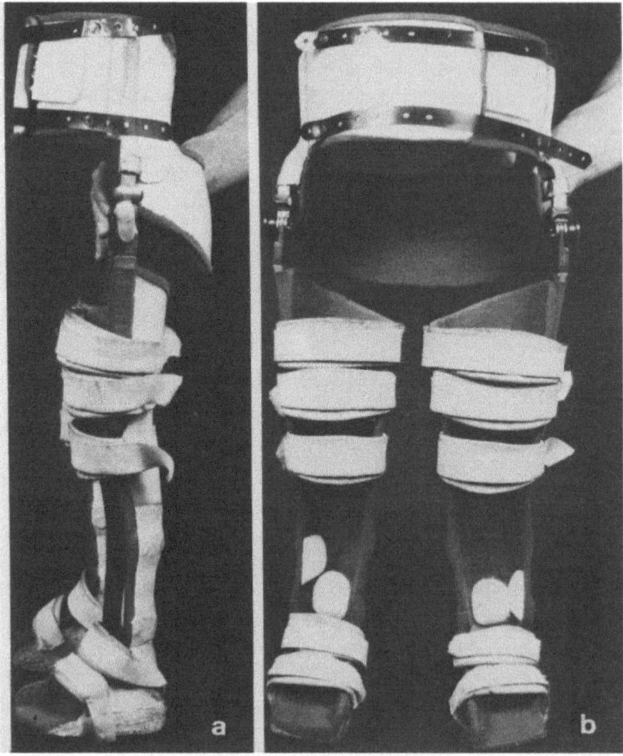

Fig. 3a and b. Myelomeningocele orthosis (hip-knee-ankle-foot-orthosis) with molded plastic shells for thigh, leg and foot, plastic trunk orthosis and hip joints with limited mobility. This orthosis is suitable for children aged 2–3 years when there is paralysis of the hip, knee and foot musculature. It allows sitting as well as standing and walking with manual help or a walker

As a rule, there is some weakness of the hip musculature in these cases. Consequently the patient finds it difficult to move the mass of the leg and orthosis. For this reason, the weight of the orthosis must be reduced as much as possible while maintaining sufficient mechanical strength. With the help of forearm crutches these patients can achieve a high degree of mobility because of their strong arm and trunk musculature. This leads to marked attrition of the orthoses.

Myelomeningocele-orthoses, i.e. hip-knee-ankle-foot-orthoses are generally necessary for lesions at the level of L3/L4 or above. In small children they can be applied with advantage as a temporary device in lesions down to L5. At the first fitting between the ages of 18 months and 3 years, a solid knee-ankle-foot-orthosis consisting of a molded shell for foot and thigh is attached by means of a Herzog-Sharrard semi-mobile hip joint to a plastic trunk orthosis (Fig. 3a, b). The lack of active hip extension is compensated for by the three-point action with anterior pressure on the distal thigh and the thorax as well as opposing pressure on the pelvis from the back. A good sitting position is possible when the hip joint lock is released. A mobility of 10° remains for extension, flexion and ab-adduction when the orthosis is locked with extended hips (Ruepp 1974), (Fig. 4a, b).

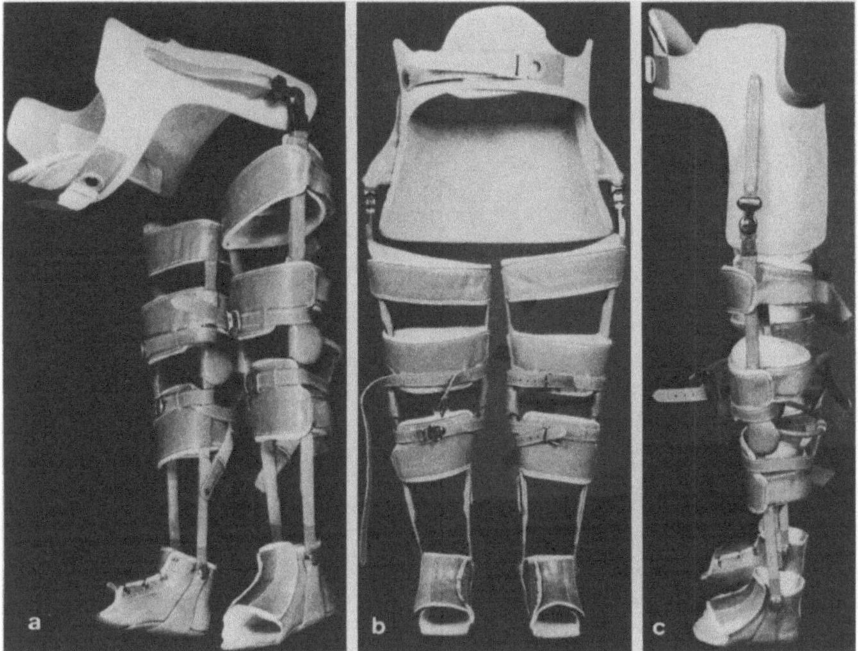

Fig. 4a–c. Hip-knee-ankle-foot orthosis with molded plastic trunk part, hip and knee joints, for use after the age of 3 when there is paralysis of the hip, knee and foot. Aim: to walk with walker or forearm crutches or even without support. It permits sitting with bent knees

To teach standing, the orthosis is first used on a tilt table which also allows balance reactions to be trained. There is enough freedom of movement in the hip joint of the orthosis to allow ambulation at a later stage. As a rule, one proceeds from walking with manual help to ambulation in parallel bars or with a rollator and finally to the use of forearm crutches with quadripedal and later monopedal gait. This orthosis has the advantage that there is relative freedom in the trunk section for torsion around the vertical axis (Fig. 3a, b/4a–c). One can assume that the torsion movements of the trunk counteract a tendency to scoliosis.

Asymmetries of paralysis in myelomeningocele patients are frequent. They render the fitting with hip-ankle-foot-orthosis more difficult and require specific measures. In order to impede progressive pelvic obliquity in connection with an adduction tendency of one hip and abduction of the contralateral side, the frontal motion of the Herzog-Sharrard hip joint must be partially blocked.

Results

An orthosis was necessary in 78% of the patients examined. Two young children had not yet been fitted at the time of follow-up and an orthosis was not necessary in 7 children. A

Table 3. Walking ability with and without orthosis in children aged 3 years and over

	Without orthosis		With orthosis	
	%	Number of children	%	Number of children
Unable to walk	56	18	3	1
Able to walk with support	31	10	75	24
Able to walk freely	13	4	22	7

hip-knee-ankle-foot-orthosis was prescribed in 15 patients, a pair of knee-ankle-foot-orthoses in 4 patients and 13 children required uni- or bilateral ankle-foot-orthoses.

Among the patients supplied with orthoses, 56% were unable to walk without them, 31% could walk with help and only 13% could walk freely but less well without apparatus.

Thanks to orthotic fitting, 79% of the children aged 3 years and over could be taught to walk. A 3 year old child who was not yet able to walk at the time of examination could stand with the help of a hip-knee-ankle-foot-orthosis (Table 3). The duration of wear of each type of orthosis is represented in Table 4. It is expected that some of the children wearing a hip-knee-ankle-foot-orthosis will be fitted with a knee-ankle-foot-orthosis with continued training.

Ankle-foot-orthosis helped 3 children to walk freely, an improvement in the gait pattern could be achieved in 9 and one child learned to walk with support.

The knee-ankle-foot-orthoses enabled one patient to walk freely, while 3 children learned to ambulate with support. Hip-knee-ankle-foot-orthoses helped 12 children

Table 4. Duration of wear of the orthosis

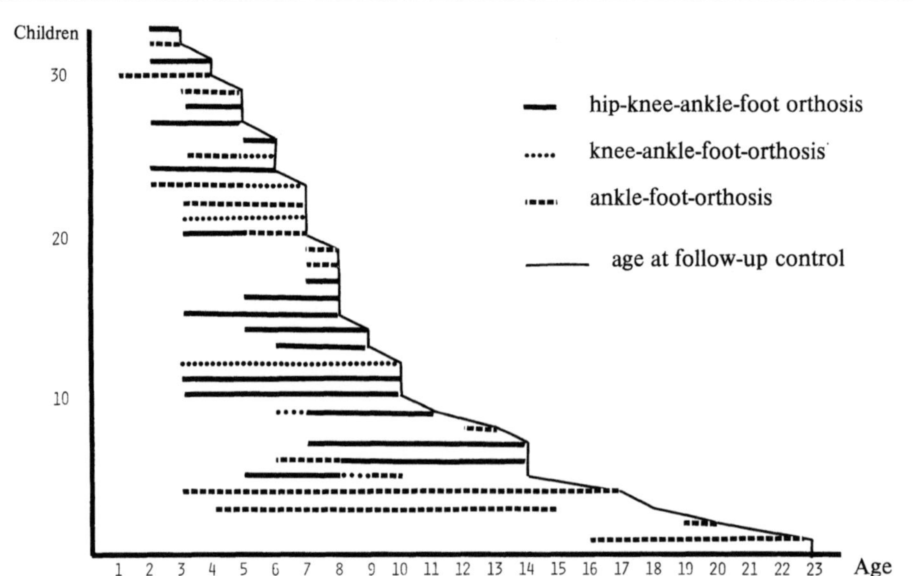

Table 5. Pathological fractures in 6 children (= 15% of the patients) with 9 fractures (= 1.5 fractures per patient)

patient	age	fracture	remarks
1	5	supracondylar fracture of the right femur	2 months after femoral derotation-varisation-osteotomy
2	5	supracondylar fracture of the right femur	3 months after acetabuloplasty
3	5	supracondylar fracture of the left femur	bedrest because of ventricular drainage dysfunction
4	3	supramalleolar fracture of the left tibia	bedrest because of pneumonia
5	5	supramalleolar fracture of the left tibia	within 2 months after Chiari pelvic osteotomy
		supramalleolar fracture of the left tibia	after Chiari pelvic osteotomy
6	4	supracondylar fracture of the left femur	within 2 months after femoral derotation-varisation osteotomy
		supramalleolar fracture of the left tibia	within 2 months after femoral derotation-varisation osteotomy of femur
		supracondylar fracture of the right femur	within 2 months after femoral derotation-varisation osteotomy

previously incapable of standing to stand and walk. Three children only able to stand could be taught to walk with such an orthosis. Six patients suffered pathological fractures (= 15%). They occurred within 2 months of prolonged bed rest following major operations or pneumonia. Two of these six patients had multiple fractures, one had 2 and the other 3 fractures (Table 5).

Discussion

Optimal orthotic fitting is of major importance for children with paralysis resulting from myelomeningocele. Independent standing and walking with or without forearm crutches can usually be achieved with time in lesions up to the lower thoracic level. This not only improves participation in daily activities but above all prevents complications such as disturbances in circulation and decubiti, as well as demineralization of bone resulting in pathological fractures and kidney stones. Contractures of the hip, knee and ankle joints as well as secondary scoliosis caused by the patients' constant tendency to sit or to be recumbent can be largely prevented. Naturally scoliosis, kyphosis and hyperlordosis due to congenital malformations of the vertebrae cannot be influenced to any major degree.

The orthosis also aids in maintaining adequate symmetrical movements of the hip joints. It contributes to the prevention of paralytic hip dislocation or reduces the number of operations necessary to avoid it. Morbidity and the number of hospitalizations can thus be reduced. For these reasons there appears to be a justifiable expense-to-efficiency relationship in spite of the relatively high cost of the orthoses including their maintenance cost.

According to statistics compiled by Tachdijan (1972), one must reckon with a pathological fracture in 25% of children with myelomeningocele. Many patients suffer multiple or recurrent fractures. Parsch and Schulitz (1972) reported an average of 2.6 fractures per child. In the patients examined here, only 15% suffered from pathological fractures; an average of 1.5 fractures per child was observed.

In 94% of our 41 patients, free or supported walking could be achieved with an adequate orthosis. Only half the children could walk without them. Two young children had not yet been provided with an orthosis at the time of examination. A 3 year old child was not yet able to walk at the time of examination.

In spite of sensory disturbances of the patient's foot and leg skin breakdown rarely occurs if there is good cooperation between parents and orthotist.

Summary

Forty one patients with myelomeningoceles between the ages of 3 and 22 years were examined with emphasis on the orthotic prescription. The orthoses used and their indications are described. Ability to stand and walk is the primary goal of this aid. Osteoporosis, occurrence of pathological fractures and appearance of flexion contractures of hips and knees can also be successfully combatted.

References

Delpierre J, Lokietek W, Rambouts JJ (1977) Le premier appareil de l'enfant paraplégique. Acta Orthop Belg 43:354

De Souza LJ, Carroll N (1976) Ambulation of the braced myelomeningocele patient. J Bone Joint Surg 58–A:1112

Drennan JC (1976) Orthotic management of the myelomeningocele spine. Dev Med Child Neurol (Suppl) 37:97

Hoffer M, Feiwell M, Perry R, Perry J, Bonnett Ch (1973) Functional ambulation in patients with myelomeningocele. J Bone Joint Surg 55–A:137

Lindseth RE, Glancy J (1974) Polypropylene lower-extremity braces for paraplaegia due to myelomeningocele. J Bone Joint Surg 56–A:556

Murdoch G (1976) The advance in orthotics. E. Arnold, London

Parsch KP, Schulitz KP (1972) Das Spina-bifida-Kind. G. Thieme, Stuttgart

Renoirte Ph, Bellen P (1977) La place des orthèses dans le traitement des séquelles du méningo-myélocèle. Acta Orthop Belg 43:345

Ruepp R (1971) Die orthetische Versorgung von Kindern bei Lähmungen der Bein- und Hüftmuskulatur. APO Rev. 10:2

Tachdjian MO (1972) Paediatric orthopedics. W.B. Saunders, Philadelphia

Translated from the German: Schürmann K, Baumann JU (1979) Konservative orthopädische Behandlungsmöglichkeiten bei Myelomeningocelen-Kindern. Orthopäde 8:350–355
© Springer Verlag 1979

List of Contributors

Baumann, Dr. J.U.
Kinderspital CH-4000 Basel, Switzerland

Judet, Dr. J.
Square Jouvenet, F-75015 Paris, France

Judet, Dr. H.
Square Jouvenet, F-75015 Paris, France

Maquet, Dr. P.
Chirurgie Orthopédique, B-4070 Aywaille 25, Thier Busset, Belgium

Schneider, Prof. Dr. R.
Regionalspital CH-2500 Biel, Switzerland

Schreiber, Prof. Dr. A.
Orthopädische Universitätsklinik Balgrist, CH-8000 Zürich, Switzerland

Schürmann, Dr. K.
Orthopädische Klinik, Chirurgisches Departement der Universität Basel, CH-4000 Basel, Switzerland

Wagner, Prof. Dr. H.
Orthopädische Klinik Wichernhaus, D-8503 Nürnberg/Altdorf, Federal Republic of Germany

Springer AV Instruction Program

Films:

Theoretical and practical bases of internal fixation, results of experimental research:

Internal Fixation – Basic Principles and Modern Means

The Biomechanics of Internal Fixation

The Ligaments of the Knee Joint Pathophysiology

Internal fixation of fractures and in corrective surgery:

Internal Fixation of Forearm Fractures

Internal Fixation of Noninfected Diaphyseal Pseudarthroses

Internal Fixation of Malleolar Fractures

Internal Fixation of Patella Fractures

Medullary Nailing

Internal Fixation of the Distal End of the Humerus

Internal Fixation of Mandibular Fractures

Corrective Osteotomy of the Distal Tibia

Internal Fixation of Tibial Head Fractures
(available in German only)

Joint replacement:

Total Hip Prostheses (3 parts)
Part 1: Instruments. Operation on Model
Part 2: Operative Technique
Part 3: Complications. Special Cases

Elbow-Arthroplasty with the New GSB-Prosthesis

Total Wrist Joint Replacement

Slide Series:

ASIF-Technique for Internal Fixation of Fractures

Manual of Internal Fixation

The Ligaments of Knee Joint – Pathophysiology
(in preparation)

Small Fragment Set Manual

Internal Fixation of Patella and Malleolar Fractures

Total Hip Prostheses
Operation on Model and in vivo, Complications and Special Cases

Asepsis in Surgery

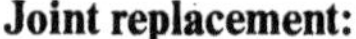

■ Further films and slide series in preparation

■ Technical data: 16 mm and super-8 (color, magnetic sound, optical sound), videocassettes. Slide series in ringbinders

■ Films in English or German, several in French; slide series with multilingual legends

■ Please ask for information material

Sales:
Springer-Verlag,
Heidelberger Platz 3,
D-1000 Berlin 33,

or

Springer-Verlag New York Inc
175 Fifth Avenue,
New York, NY 10010

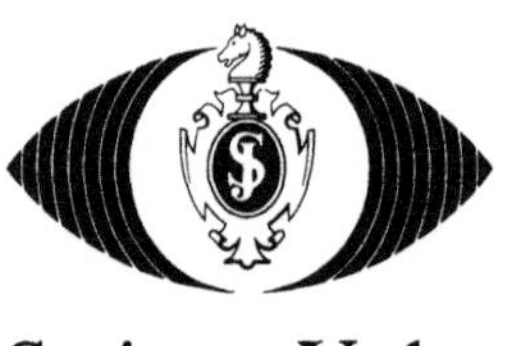

Springer-Verlag
Berlin
Heidelberg
New York